SURVIVING BIOTERRORISM

Natural and Medical Remedies for Biological, Chemical and Nuclear Attack

From the Editors of
The Doctors' Prescription for Healthy Living

This information is for educational purposes only. It is intended to help in the event of biological and chemical weapons attacks on civilian populations. It is not provided in order to diagnose or treat any disease, illness, or injury of the body, mind, or spirit.

The author, publisher, and distributors of this work accept no responsibility for people using or misusing the potentially life-saving information in this text.

ISBN 1-893910-25-3
Printed in Canada
Published by Freedom Press
1801 Chart Trail
Topanga, CA 90290
Bulk Orders Available: (800) 959-9797
E-mail: info@freedompressonline.com

Cover/Book Design by Bonnie Lambert

"The Martians had no resistance to the bacteria in our atmosphere to which we have long become immune....After all that men could do had failed, the Martians were destroyed and the world was saved by the littlest things which God in his wisdom had put on the Earth."

— Concluding narration
of the 1952 movie version
of *The War of the Worlds*

"Know the enemy and know yourself, and in a hundred battles you will never be in peril."

— Sun Tzu

Table of Contents

Introduction *7*

CHAPTER 1 Biological and Chemical Warfare FAQs *11*

CHAPTER 2 Protecting Against Nerve Agents *32*

CHAPTER 3 Protecting Against Biological Weapons *58*

CHAPTER 4 Nutritional Protection Against Bioterrorism *102*

CHAPTER 5 Nuclear and Radiation Protection *144*

CHAPTER 6 Protection Measures Recommended by the Department of Homland Security *174*

CHAPTER 7 Preparing for Biological and Chemical Terrorism: A Practical Guide to Antibiotics and Their Usage for Survival *198*

Notes *223*

Introduction

The likelihood that biological, chemical, radiological or nuclear weapons will cause panic among civilian decreases when we become better educated regarding these threats and we feel some measure of self-control.

We hope that this guide will never be needed. But events of September 11, 2001 and subsequent events have shown us that the global environment is a rapidly changing scene. Worldwide changes in natural, political, social, and economic paradigms result in security risks which confront us all, no matter where we are located geographically.

Minimizing these risks and fighting against panic and hysteria requires knowledge and planning. The purpose of ***SURVIVING BIOTERRORISM—Natural and Medical Remedies for Biological, Chemical and Nuclear Attack*** is to assist individuals, corporations, and health-care professionals with a quick reference guide to self-protection in such instances.

Advance risk management planning combined with current information on self-protection is the most effective way to defend yourself and loved ones against terrorism.

The philosophy of this guide is that risk management through preparedness and education is the true way to maximizing personal safety—given all of the circumstances and understanding that some events are out of our individual control to stop or influence.

Until recently, we in the United States have not given much thought to the specter of chemical and biological warfare. Our fathers and grandfathers who fought in World War I are almost all gone now, and the poet's image of gassed soldiers fumbling for their helmets has been considered merely a historical footnote—if it is remembered at all. But forgetting is a luxury we can no longer afford.

Nothing has changed except the increased availability of chemical and biological weapons; now more than ever we must be able to both defend against attack and manage chemical, biological, and radiological casualties.

The good news is that the development of passive countermeasures for chemical and biological defense (pretreatments, therapies, timely detectors, effective protective equipment, and protective foods and nutritional supplements) can help to make us stronger and significantly reduce the magnitude of this threat and, with proper preparation, even make it manageable. Of course, proactive countermeasures involving our federal, state, and local security agencies are also essential.

In the meantime, we can educate ourselves on self-protection at minimal cost and with great potential benefit. One of the reasons that chemical and biological weapons are considered so dangerous is that in daily clinical practice, health professionals hardly ever see patients whose conditions have any similarity to casualties of chemical and some of the more exotic biological agents.

This guidebook focuses on self-protection. Its publication may be even more timely than we had expected, especially considering the increased threat of terrorism—both foreign and domestic. Terrorist attacks at home and abroad have heightened the interest of civilian health-care providers and first-responders and of other governmental agencies such as the Federal Emergency Management Agency and the Public Health Service that would be required to respond in case of an attack on our own soil, as well as typical everyday persons who simply wish to be better informed about potential threats and what they can do about them. Both military and nonmilitary healthcare providers will also find this guide to be extremely useful.

The scientists from whom this information has been compiled are recognized worldwide as the foremost experts in the medical aspects of chemical and biological warfare. Their overriding goal is this: to understand the threats of chemical, biological, and radiological weapons and how to respond to them, and, by understanding the threats, sustain fewer casualties. If you are prepared, you will survive in most cases of terrorism. As a nation, preparation and self-protection provide us with strength and confidence to go about our daily lives, living in freedom.

CHAPTER ONE

Biological and Chemical Warfare FAQs

"Gas! Gas!" This warning cry, so common in World War I, almost became real to U.S. forces again as they prepared to liberate Kuwait in late 1990. The threat of chemical, and even biological, warfare was foremost in the minds of U.S. military personnel during Operation Desert Shield, the preparation for the Persian Gulf War.

Iraq was known to have a large stockpile of chemical weapons and had demonstrated during its conflict with Iran that it would use them. It was not until after the Persian Gulf War that the United Nations Special Commission on Iraq confirmed that Saddam Hussein also had biological agents loaded in weapons. The chemical and biological threats were major concerns to those in the military medical departments who would be called on to care for poisoned or infected casualties, possibly in a chemically contaminated environment. Fortunately the ground war of the Persian Gulf War (Operation Desert Storm) was brief, and even more fortunately, our adversary did not employ these weapons.

In the desert during the fall and winter of 1990–1991, the threat of chemical warfare became very real to our military medical personnel. The threat of biological warfare was no less feared. The military medical departments realized that medical personnel were not prepared to provide care to chemical or biological casualties or to function in a contaminated environment. We now know that, for the most part, our civilian population is even less prepared. But this guide will help us to prepare.

Hundreds of thousands of troops were supplied with chemical pretreatment and therapeutic agents and thousands were immunized against anthrax and the botulinum toxins, the two most likely biological battlefield threats.

Two lessons were learned from this conflict, lessons that should never be forgotten. The first was that there are countries that have chemical and biological weapons, and there are other countries and terrorist groups that might obtain or produce them. The second was that we must be prepared at all times. As long as potential adversaries exist, the United States is likely to face a chemical or biological battlefield.

Medical personnel of the United States have not treated a chemical casualty on the battlefield for nearly eight decades, and they have never treated a biological casualty. Chemical agents have not been used as weapons in a major war or in any military conflict in which the United States has been involved since World War I. Despite the recent dissolution of the Warsaw Pact, the breakup of the Soviet Union, and other events that have seemingly reduced the conventional military threat to the United States, a textbook for medical personnel on the management of chemical and biological agent casualties is still urgently needed.

The breakup of the Soviet Union and the consequent glut of biowarfare experts on the world employment market, combined with destitute or poorly paid scientists and officials who may be willing to sell such weapons or their secrets at the "right price," may have actually increased the threat of biological proliferation.

Recent Targets of Chemical or Biological Agents

- Laos (mid to late 1970s; alleged)
- Kampuchea (late 1970s and early 1980s; alleged)
- Afghanistan (1980s; alleged)
- Iran (1980s; Iran–Iraq War; confirmed)
- Iraqi Kurds (1988; confirmed)

When has biological and chemical warfare been used before?

During the Arab–Israeli War (also called the Yom Kippur War) of 1973, chemical weapons were not used. While processing captured soldiers, however, Israeli troops found that the Egyptians carried personal protective equipment, decontamination kits containing items unfamiliar to U.S. personnel, and an antidote with which we were also unfamiliar. This evidence suggested that the Egyptians were prepared for a chemical battlefield, and the components of the antidote suggested that they were prepared for the use of the nerve agent soman. The U.S. military soon issued the antidote to U.S. troops, only to withdraw it about five years later.

In the mid to late 1970s, reports began to appear that chemicals were being used against Hmong tribesmen in Laos. The Hmong had been loyal to the United States and had served this country in many ways during the Vietnam War; it was suggested that chemicals were being used against the Hmong in retaliation. Investigations were conducted by U.S. State Department personnel, by a medical team sent by the U.S. Army Surgeon General, and by international groups. Little definitive evidence was discovered, primarily because the alleged attacks took place deep in Laos. The victims took weeks to travel to Thailand to be examined, and outsiders could not enter Laos to examine the attack sites. The Hmong who reached Thailand provided graphic accounts of attacks by sprays and bombs from airplanes and how these "smokes," which were of all colors, killed many in their villages. One member of the medical team brought back a sample of a yellow substance on the outer (barklike) layers of a bamboo culm (i.e., stalk); the sample had been given to him by a Hmong, who claimed that the material had killed many of his fellow villagers. This yellow substance, along with samples from many other locations, later became known as "yellow rain."

Moreover, in the late 1970s and early 1980s, allegations were made of chemical agent use against refugees fleeing the barbaric conditions that existed in Kampuchea at that time. The clinical response of the exposed humans did not fit what we understood about the effects of classic chemical agents. Tearing and itching looked like the effects of tear gas. Convulsions suggested nerve agents. But the occurrence of internal hemorrhage and skin lesions could not be explained. Analysis of a leaf sample collected in Kampuchea 24 hours after an attack implicated trichothecene mycotoxins, a family of toxins produced by fungi but having characteristics more like chemical than biological agents.

If mycotoxins were in fact used, it was the first recorded use of biological agents since before World

War II, when the Japanese used them against the Chinese in the early 1940s.

In the 1980s, Soviet troops battled Afghan rebels protesting the communist Afghan regime. During this lengthy conflict, frequent allegations were made of the use of chemical agents against the Afghans. One of these chemicals, known as BlueX, was said to cause instant immobilization, the victim remaining in place for a number of hours before recovering. The use of other, more lethal agents was also alleged, but again no definitive evidence was found.

The most widespread and most open use of chemical weapons on a battlefield in recent decades was by Iraq in its conflict with Iran. This time the evidence of chemical use was conclusive. Undetonated shells were sampled and their contents were analyzed by several laboratories in Europe. A vesicant or blister agent (mustard) and a nerve agent (tabun) were identified. About 100 Iranian soldiers with chemical wounds were sent to European hospitals for care; their wounds were consistent with vesicant (mustard) injury. A team appointed by the U.N. secretariat went to Iranian battlefields and hospitals and found chemical shells and patients with chemical injuries. The public outcry at the use of these weapons was less than overwhelming. Ignoring protests from the world community, Iraq continued to use these agents.

Evacuating wounded soldiers to Europe not only lessened the burden on the medical facilities in Iran (although the number sent was a small fraction of the total) and provided soldiers with good medical care, but it also provided the rest of the world with evidence that Iraq was using these weapons. In general, the casualties were sent privately, not through governmental connections. Physicians in Europe accepted the patients and assumed responsibility for their care, usually in private hospitals (a situation that made a retrospective analysis of the care rendered and the effectiveness of different treatment regimens difficult).

A similar situation enabled three physicians from the U.S. Army medical community to examine several casualties from Iraq's use of chemical weapons.

On March 19, 1988, Iraqi airplanes bombed the village of Halabja in Iraq. The inhabitants were Kurdish Iraqi citizens, a tribespeople who live in the region where the borders of Turkey, Iran, and Iraq meet. The casualties from this raid received worldwide media attention. The chemical weapons allegedly used were nerve agents, cyanide, and mustard. The casualties were cared for by Iran, and five of them (a man, a woman, and three young children, all unrelated) were sent to the United States for care by an Iranian physician living here. On examination, the casualties were found to have skin lesions and pulmonary pathological changes (as determined by radiograph) consistent with mustard exposure.

Other items in the news over the past decade have suggested that the proliferation of chemical and biological agents is greater than we might hope. For example, numerous accounts claimed that Libya had built a facility capable of chemical agent production at Rabta—Libya's protestation that this facility was a pharmaceutical plant notwithstanding. One report even noted that monthly production was about 30 tons of mustard.

In 1979, an accident at a previously undetected biological weapons plant in Sverdlovsk, Russia, surprised even the intelligence community. At least 66 people living or working downwind of the plant died of pulmonary anthrax. Soviet troops quickly attempted to decontaminate the facility and the city following an airborne release of anthrax spores and medical teams instituted preventive therapy, but the message was clear. The Soviet biological warfare program was thriving, more than six years after the Soviet Union had signed the Biological Weapons Convention.

In addition to their being used on the battlefield, chemical and biological agents might also be used in terrorist attacks. The nerve agent sarin was twice used in Japan. The first incident, in Matsumoto in June 1994, produced more than 200 casualties, including seven fatalities. In the second incident—in the Tokyo subway system on March 20, 1995—5,510 people were taken to medical facilities or sought medical assistance. About 20 percent of these were hospitalized, and 12 died. The cult that was accused of both attacks was found to have a large facility for manufacturing both chemical and biological agents. This shows us that it could happen in other nations as well.

In the face of overwhelming evidence, the former Soviet Union continued to officially deny having an offensive biological weapons program until 1992, when Russian president Boris Yeltsin admitted publicly to having maintained a program until March of that year. Since then, visits by teams from the United States and the United Kingdom to former biological warfare facilities under the Joint United States/United Kingdom/Russia Trilateral Statement on Biological Weapons have clearly documented the capabilities to produce biological warfare agents in massive quantities.

Verification of compliance with agreements such as the Trilateral and with the chemical and biological weapons conventions are plagued by the "dual-use" nature of the facilities in which these agents are developed and produced. A legitimate chemical facility can be converted fairly easily for the manufacture of chemical agents. On threat of inspection by an international group, the facility can readily be converted back to a legitimate use. The dual-use nature of production facilities is even more applicable to the production of biological agents. Partly for this reason, chemical and biological weapons have been called "the poor man's atom bomb." It has also been said that agents can be made in a bathtub, which may be true to a limited

FYI: Differences between Chemical and Biological Agents

Chemical and biological agents differ in several important ways. Chemical agents are typically man-made through the use of industrial chemical processes.

Biological agents are either replicating agents (bacteria or viruses) or nonreplicating materials (toxins or physiologically active proteins or peptides) that can be produced by living organisms.

Some of the nonreplicating biological agents can also be produced through either chemical synthesis, solid phase protein synthesis, or recombinant expression methods. Almost none of the biological agents are dermally active (the mycotoxins are a rare exception) and none are volatile. On the other hand, most of the chemical agents are dermally active, volatile, or both.

Therefore, while many of the dermally active or volatile chemical agents can be disseminated as liquids or aerosols, the biological agents must be dispersed as respirable aerosols (particles approximately 1–10 μm in diameter). Dispersing a respirable aerosol among civilians requires a high-energy generating system to produce the small particle size, appropriate weather conditions to assure that the aerosol cloud stays near the ground, and adequate infectivity or toxicity of the agent to produce the desired effect. Except for infectivity, these are all important practical requirements for the field use of chemical, as well as biological, warfare agents.

extent for a skilled microbiologist or chemist. Production of even tactical quantities of these agents and their deployment on the battlefield, however, is not a trivial undertaking.

What are chemical agents?

All chemical agents are relatively easy to synthesize, do not require sophisticated missiles, bombs, or other delivery devices for dispersion through populations and, unlike most biological agents, are capable of producing illness rapidly. Many of these agents are "weapons of opportunity" confiscated from industry or transport vehicles rather than manufactured by terrorists.

Nerve agents are highly toxic; as little as one milligram (mg) can be lethal to an adult. Most nerve agents are highly volatile and are designed to produce gas clouds that are inhaled by victims. Sarin, in addition to being volatile, has a vapor density 4.86 times that of water, which makes it easier to breathe by children because it is concentrated closer to the ground.

Mustard gas, ammonia, and chlorine are corrosive chemicals that may be used in a chemical-biological incident. They are designed to injure skin, eyes, and nasal mucosa, producing severe pain and incapacitation. If these chemicals are inhaled, life-threatening pneumonitis may also occur. With agents such as these, skin decontamination by showering is the mainstay of therapy. Pulmonary support, including intubation and mechanical ventilation, may be necessary for those with severe pulmonary injury.

Other chemical agents are designed to incapacitate rather than kill. However, particularly in victims with significant chronic illness, the incapacitating agents can result in life-threatening toxicity.

What are biological agents?

Biological weapons are referred to as a "poor man's nuclear bomb" because they are easy to manufacture, can be deployed without sophisticated delivery systems, and have the ability to kill or injure hundreds of thousands of people. Simple devices such as crop-dusting airplanes, small perfume atomizers, or even mail letters are effective delivery systems for biological agents.

In contrast to chemical, conventional, and nuclear weapons that generate immediate effects, biological agents are generally associated with a delay in the onset of illness (hours to days). Moreover, illnesses from biological weapons are likely to be unrecognized in their initial stages. With highly transmissible agents (e.g., plague and smallpox), the time delay in recognition can result in widespread secondary exposure to others, including health-care personnel. Depending on the communicability of the microbe, wide geographic paths can be affected when infected individuals who are asymptomatic travel by airplane to other parts of the country or world.

Biological weapon releases on civilian populations have also occurred in the recent past. In 1984 in Oregon, approximately 750 people experienced salmonellosis after bacteria were spread on salad bars in an effort to disrupt local elections. An inadvertent release of anthrax in April 1979 by a military facility in Sverdlovsk, in the former Soviet republic, produced mass infection as distant as 50 kilometers, with 66 documented deaths.

Biological agents include bacteria, viruses, or preformed toxins, and, for most, quantities as small as one kilogram (kg, the equivalent of 2.2 pounds) can injure or kill thousands of people. Marked diversity exists in the type of injury produced by infectious agents, with toxic effects ranging from incapacitation to death.

Anthrax has been extensively developed as a biological weapon and, as we now know, is considered the most likely candidate for a biological release. The causative organism, *Bacillus anthracis*, is a Gram-positive sporulating rod. Because its initial symptoms are nonspecific and experience with the disease is uncommon, anthrax may be misdiagnosed. The first indication of an aerosol exposure may be groups of patients with severe influenza-like disease and a high case-fatality rate. After a few hours or days and the possible appearance of improvement in affected individuals, progression to fever, dyspnea (i.e., shortness of breath), and shock occurs. Human-to-human transmission of anthrax does not occur.

Plague, caused by *Yersinia pestis*, is also considered a potential bacterial weapon. Unlike anthrax, pneumonic plague can be highly contagious, quickly infecting families or health-care professionals. Untreated, plague carries a mortality as high as 100 percent.

Other bacterial agents with high potential for use as biologic weapons are *Brucella species* (brucellosis), *Coxiella burnetii* (Q fever), and *Francisella tularensis* (tularemia).

Viruses of concern include variola (smallpox), Ebola, and other hemorrhagic viruses and the viral encephalitides. Because smallpox was eradicated globally in 1980, and children are no longer being immunized, more than 80 percent of the adult population and 100 percent of children are susceptible to the virus. Smallpox produces a characteristic centrifugal rash consisting of vesicles with umbilicated centers. The rash, once familiar to clinicians, is now unlikely to be recognized quickly and can be mistaken for varicella. Reported mortality from smallpox ranges from 3 percent to 30 percent, respectively, in individuals who have or have not been immunized.

Toxins derived from biological agents generally have the characteristics of chemical agents, producing illness within hours of exposure. These agents are not infectious. Botulinum toxin, one of the most potent toxins known, can be extracted from the bacterium *Clostridium botulinum*; highly potent, it is 100,000 times more toxic than sarin. Within one to three days of exposure, victims experience cranial nerve disturbances followed by descending paralysis and respiratory failure.

The enterotoxin of *Staphylococcus aureus* is also incapacitating, although not highly lethal, except in those at extremes of age or with chronic illness. Exposure to this toxin can produce severe diarrhea that results in marked fluid losses and frank shock.

Ricin and aflatoxin are plant-derived toxins. Ricin, a potent toxin obtained from *Ricinus communis*, the castor bean, was developed as a chemotherapy agent but has been used in assassinations. Inhalation of ricin produces weakness, fever, cough, and pulmonary edema within 24 hours, with death from hypoxemia occurring in 36 to 72 hours. When ingested, ricin produces severe vomiting and diarrhea, resulting in cardiovascular collapse. Treatment is supportive; there is no antidote.

How can we be exposed to chemical or biological agents?

Acts of chemical-biological terrorism use various routes of exposure. Inhaled airborne agents may produce toxicity by introducing infection via the respiratory tract (e.g., anthrax, smallpox), by producing lung injury (e.g., chlorine), or by their absorption with resulting systemic effects (e.g., cyanide). Aerosolized agents may also be designed to produce skin injury (e.g., vesicants, corrosives). Finally, aerosolized agents can be designed for absorption through the skin with resulting systemic effects (e.g., VX and other viscous nerve agents).

Ingestion of contaminated food or water is another important route of exposure. Many biological agents are efficiently introduced via this route. For example, as few as 100 *Shigella dysenteriae* bacteria can produce severe bacterial enteritis.

Early signs and symptoms of illness from chemical or biological weapons are often unrecognized by health-care professionals. For example, mild exposure to nerve agents may produce only nausea, vomiting, and weakness. Many biological agents initially cause only fever or a flulike illness.

Are there environmental consequences when chemical or biological toxins are released?

The environmental toll of a chemical or biological toxin release can be comparable to that from nuclear fallout. Depending on the agent, local areas can become uninhabitable for days to months. In the case of anthrax, the ability of the bacterium to sporulate can result in soil contamination by spores that remain viable for more than 30 years. Viscous nerve agents such as VX also have significant environmental persistence, leading to area contamination that prevents families from returning to their homes.

What are the signs that a poison gas attack (or a chemical accident) might be taking place?

One of the many unsettling characteristics of chemical agents is that some of them cannot be seen or smelled. Citizens can protect themselves by observing the following rule of thumb: If a single person is on the ground, choking or seizing, it is likely this individual is having a heart attack or some sort of seizure. However, if several people are down, coughing, vomiting, or seizing, they could be reacting to the presence of a toxic substance. Evacuate the area immediately and dial 911, making sure to tell the dispatcher that a hazardous gas may be present.

If indoors, exit the building as rapidly as possible. Once outside, if you believe that you may have been exposed to the toxic substance, discarding your modesty and shedding your clothes could save your life. Taking off your outer clothing can remove roughly 80 percent of the contamination hazard. Look for a nearby fountain, pool, or other source of water and jump in so that you can quickly and thoroughly rinse any skin that may have been exposed. Studies show that water alone is an effective decontaminant.

Rescuers will arrive within minutes, and firefighters will hook up hoses and spray everyone to decontaminate them. Try to remain calm. Rescuers will triage everyone so that they can give medical attention to the most seriously affected individuals first. Even if you are showing no symptoms of exposure (e.g., eye problems), paramedics and physicians on scene will want to give you a checkup and advise you about followup care. Police officers will also want to speak with you about what you may have observed that could help them catch the individual(s) responsible.

If outdoors, birds and other small animals would very quickly be overcome by a poison gas, so if birds are dropping from the sky, that is another warning sign of toxic trouble. The most important thing to do is to get a physical barrier between you and the toxic cloud. Get indoors quickly; preferably you should go into a building, but even being inside a car will help. Shut all windows and doors and turn off the air conditioner. Try to plug any air drafts (e.g., under doors). This technique is known as sheltering in place. Call 911 and notify authorities that a hazardous gas may be present. If that is indeed the case, the wind will carry the toxic hazard away within a relatively short period of time. Stay indoors and turn on the television and/or radio for news and announcements. Authorities will notify you when it is safe to go outside. If you are at home, put your clothes in a plastic bag and take a shower, which will help remove any contamination that might have occurred before you were able to get indoors.

Should citizens buy gas masks?

The chances that terrorists will turn to poisonous substances instead of conventional bombs are very, very remote. However, if it makes you feel better to purchase a gas mask, by all means, go ahead. We especially recommend gas masks be carried by anyone riding the subways of Washington, D.C., New York, and other east coast cities. The odds are 99.9 percent you will never need to use it, but, in the event of such an attack, having a gas mask in your briefcase might well save your life. Please make sure that you are properly fitted, as a loose gas mask defeats the purpose. Also, please ensure that you are properly instructed in the use of the mask.

Note also that the only nation that has ever issued gas masks to all of its citizens is Israel.

What are the signs of a biological attack?

The media has repeatedly broadcast that biological agents can be dispersed from commercial sprayers, such as crop dusters. Often omitted from these reports is the fact that, among other complications, commercial equipment would have to be modified for such an attack strategy to have a chance of success.

Still, crop dusters are out of place over cities, and the FBI has already placed restrictions about where they can fly. Were the authors to see one over a metropolitan area, they would immediately go indoors, shut all windows and doors, turn off the air conditioner, and notify authorities. The same would hold true for any other unusual spraying activities. For instance, a person tending a roof-top garden would not raise my suspicions, but an individual deliberately spraying a substance from a rooftop, or a truck dispersing a misty substance through side vents, would.

Keep in mind that occasionally local authorities employ helicopters and other means to spray approved pesticides to control mosquitoes and other pests. Officially sanctioned spraying activities are announced well in advance, repeatedly. A call to local authorities can confirm whether any spraying that you might observe would fall into that category.

What precautions can citizens take with their water supply?

Poisoning a city's water supply is much more easily said than done. However, citizens can protect themselves by boiling their drinking water, which will kill any microorganisms that may have survived the municipal filtration systems. Another option is to use a personal water filtration system. This will help to eliminate many types of chemical toxins. Be sure your system combines reverse osmosis with activated carbon and several types of prefilters.

CHAPTER TWO

Protecting Against Nerve Agents

Nerve agents are extremely toxic chemicals that were first developed in secrecy before and during World War II primarily for military use. Related substances are used in medicine, in pharmacology, and for other purposes, such as insecticides, but they lack the potency of the military agents. Much of the basic knowledge about the clinical effects of nerve agents comes from research performed in the decades immediately following World War II. The military stockpiles of several major powers are known to include nerve agents, and the armamentaria of other countries, as well as terrorists, are thought to have access to them.

Five organophosphorus compounds are generally regarded as nerve agents. They are commonly known as **tabun** (North Atlantic Treaty Organization [NATO] military designation, GA), **sarin** (GB), and

soman (GD); and **GF** and **VX** (also NATO military designations; these compounds have no common names). The agents in the "G" series allegedly were given the code letter G because they originated in Germany; the "V" allegedly stands for venomous. GF is an old agent, previously discarded by the United States as being of no interest. During the Persian Gulf War, it was believed that Iraq might have GF in its arsenal; however, interest has waned again and GF has retreated to obscurity.

It is very possible that nerve agents will be used in the United States as a means of terrorizing the civilian population. Most likely, such uses will be in highly populated urban centers, sporting events, large office buildings (via the ventilation system), subway systems, and possibly even airliners. It is possible to survive a nerve-gas attack if one is properly outfitted with a survival kit as is frequently distributed to military personnel. Although a recommendation for such kits is not universal, people who live in high-risk urban centers, utilize mass transit, or otherwise may be at high risk may want to consider keeping such kits in their possession or nearby.

BRIEF HISTORY OF NERVE AGENTS

The German company I. G. Farbenindustrie developed an interest in organophosphorus compounds as insecticides. On December 23, 1936, Gerhard Schrader, who headed the company's research effort, synthesized what today is known as tabun.

Over a year later, Schrader synthesized a second organophosphorus compound and named it sarin in honor of those who were instrumental in its development and production: Schrader, Ambros, Rudriger, and van der Linde.

Because the German Ministry of Defense required that substances passing certain toxicity tests be submitted to the government for further investigation, these compounds were examined for possible military use.

The potential of tabun and sarin as weapons was soon realized. A large production facility was built in Dyhernfurth and production of tabun was begun in 1942. Sarin was also produced in Dyhernfurth and possibly at another plant in Falkenhagen.

Late in World War II, Soviet troops captured the Dyhernfurth facility (then in Germany, now in Poland), dismantled it, and moved it, along with key personnel, to the former Soviet Union, where production of the agents commenced in 1946.

About 10,000 to 30,000 tons of tabun and smaller

quantities of sarin were produced and put into munitions by the Germans during World War II, but these weapons were never used.

Why they were not remains a matter of conjecture. In the waning days of World War II, troops of the United States and the United Kingdom captured some of these munitions, which were being stored at Raubkammer, a German testing facility. The munitions, which contained an agent unknown to scientists in the United Kingdom and the United States, were taken to the two countries for examination.

Over a single weekend, a small group of scientists at the UK Chemical Defence Establishment, working despite miosis (excess smallness or contraction of the pupil of the eye) caused by accidental exposure to the agent vapor, elucidated the pharmacology and toxicity of tabun and documented the antidotal activity of atropine. Thus, during the latter part of World War II, Germany possessed chemical weapons against which its foes had little protection and no antidotes.

Use of these weapons probably would have been devastating and might have altered the outcome of that conflict. The Germans had tested nerve agents on concentration camp prisoners, not only to investigate their intoxicating effects but also to develop antidotes. Many casualties, including some fatalities, were reported among the plant workers at

Dyhernfurth; the medical staff there eventually developed antidotal compounds. The Allies were unaware of these German experiments until the close of the war, months after the initial UK studies.

Soman was synthesized in 1944 by Richard Kuhn of Germany, again in a search for insecticides. Small amounts were produced, but development had not proceeded far by the end of the war. The nerve agent VX was first synthesized by an industrial concern in the United Kingdom in the early 1950s and was given to the United States for military development.

Other potential nerve agents were synthesized by scientists in the United States and United Kingdom but were not developed for military use. For example, GF, which may have been first synthesized about 1949 by a chemist in another country in the search for other nerve agents, was studied in both the United States and the United Kingdom. It was then discarded for reasons that are not entirely clear. Possibly it was too expensive to manufacture or there was no perceived need for an agent with its properties. The manufacturing process for GF is apparently similar to that for GB. During the Persian Gulf War (1990–1991), Iraq was believed to have switched from the manufacture of GB to the manufacture of GF when the precursors of GB, but not those of GF, were embargoed. The United States began to produce sarin in the early 1950s and VX in the early 1960s for potential military use; production continued for about a decade.

Sarin has also been used in terrorist attacks. In June 1994, members of a Japanese cult released sarin in an apartment complex in Matsumoto, Japan. Although there were almost 300 casualties, including seven dead, this event was not well publicized. On March 20, 1995, sarin was released on Tokyo subways. More than 5,500 people sought medical care; about 4,000 had no effects from the agent, but 12 casualties died. This incident required a major expenditure of medical resources to triage and care for the casualties.

HOW NERVE AGENTS WORK

Nerve agents are compounds that exert their biological effects by inhibition of the enzyme acetylcholinesterase (AChE). The enzyme AChE, found at the receptor sites of nerve tissue, breaks down acetylcholine very rapidly. If AChE is inhibited, the result is a build-up of acetylcholine, resulting in spasms, paralysis, and eventual death.

SYMPTOMS OF NERVE AGENT POISONING

The effects produced by nerve agent vapor begin in seconds to minutes after the onset of exposure, depending on the concentration of vapor. These effects usually reach maximal severity within minutes after the individual is removed from or protected from the vapor or may continue to worsen if the exposure continues. There is no delay in onset as there is after liquid exposure. At low exposures, the eyes, nose, airways, or a combination of these organs are usually affected. The eyes and nose are the most sensitive organs; one eye may be affected differently than the other.

High-risk Situations for Nerve Gas Attacks

- Major multinational office buildings
- Subways
- Airliners
- Buses
- Trains
- Crowded indoor events such asconcerts and sporting matches

As exposure increases slightly, the triad of eye, nose, and lung involvement is usually seen. The casualty may or may not notice dim vision and may complain of "tightness in the chest;" the latter symptom may occur in the absence of physical findings. At higher exposures, the effects in these organs intensify. Marked miosis, copious secretions from the nose and mouth, and signs of moderate to severe impairment of ventilation are seen. The casualty will complain of mild to severe dyspnea, be gasping for air, and will have obvious secretions.

The principles of treatment of nerve agent poisoning are the same as they are for any toxic substance exposure: namely, terminate the exposure; establish or maintain ventilation; administer an antidote, if one is available; and correct cardiovascular abnormalities.

GAS MASKS

The standard M40 (or M17A2) protective mask will protect against any likely field concentration of nerve agent vapor for days. It is available through select channels, probably Army-Navy surplus-type stores and survivalist equipment outfitters. The M40/M17A2 protective mask is designed to protect the wearer from field concentrations of all known chemical, biological, and riot-control agents. When worn correctly, the mask will protect the face, eyes, and respiratory tract. Wearing the ABC-M6A2 Hood attached to the M17A2 mask further protects the head, neck, and shoulder areas.

The protective mask contains two M13A2 Filter Elements. Filtration through these elements involves two separate but complementary mechanisms: (1) impaction and adsorption of agent molecules onto ASC Whetlerite carbon filtration media and (2) impaction on a high-efficiency particulate air filter paper of particles with an average diameter of 0.3 microns.

Maintenance, and, when necessary, replacement of the crucial filter elements, are of the utmost priority. The filters must be replaced whenever any of the following occurs:

- The elements are immersed in water.
- The elements are crushed, cut, or otherwise damaged.
- Excessive breathing resistance is encountered.
- Thirty days elapse in the combat theater of operations (the filters must be replaced every 30 days).

Sources: Simply enter key words "M40M17A2 protective mask" on an Internet search engine. Many companies can be found offering this equipment.

Important: Pocket-sized masks intended for victim rescue and self-rescue during chemical and biological incidents are available from several manufacturers (for example, Fume Free, Essex, Giat). One system uses layers of activated charcoal cloth to remove chemical toxicants and a particulate element for particle removal. Testing has shown the system to be effective against nerve agent simulant, hydrogen cyanide, and tear gas. The one-size fits all mask uses a hood design with a neck seal.

Important: You might want to obtain either a regular or pocket-sized gas mask if you use our subway systems or are in other high-risk situations. Again, chances are you will never need it. But on the remote chance of a nerve agent attack, you will survive. One source for such masks is located at www.investigations.com. The toll-free number is (800) 777-9366.

DECONTAMINATING YOUR SKIN

Because of the potency of liquid nerve agents and the rapidly occurring tissue damage caused by vesicants, you should be able to effectively decontaminate of all exposed skin automatically.

Decontamination Kit M291 is particularly recommended. The introduction of this kit marks a new approach to skin decontamination. The kit consists of six identical packets, each containing a mixture of activated resins. This resin mixture both adsorbs liquid chemical agents present on the victim's skin and neutralizes agents. The mixture consists of an adsorbent resin, a resin containing sulfonic acid, and a hydroxylamine-containing resin. After masking, the user opens any packet from the kit, removes the applicator pad, and applies an even coating of resin powder while scrubbing the entire skin area suspected to be contaminated. One applicator pad will decontaminate both hands and the face, if necessary. If the face must be decontaminated, then the neck (including the throat area) and the ears must also be decontaminated using a second applicator pad.

The black resin powder residue will provide a visual confirmation of the thoroughness of application and will not cause any skin irritation even after prolonged contact with skin. However, normal precau-

Self-Protection Tip:

A solution that releases chlorine, such as household bleach (5% sodium hypochlorite) or a solution that is sufficiently alkaline to neutralize the agent, such as dilute hydroxide, can also be used for physical removal and chemical neutralization of a chemical agent. Because of the potential for skin damage from 5% hypochlorite, the current military procedure is to use 0.5% hypochlorite for skin decontamination. That means 10 parts water to one part bleach. Also, if exposed, remove your clothing.

tions must be observed so that the powder does not enter open wounds, the mouth, or the eyes. One source for these kits is www.citizensafe.com.

Water is also a decontaminant since, when used in large amounts, it physically removes and dilutes chemical agents. (Most agents hydrolyze to some degree in water, but hydrolysis usually takes hours to days.) If used alone, water is not ideal; however, if nothing else is available, flushing with large amounts of water to physically remove the chemical agent is satisfactory. Water should be used to wash off other decontaminants. Commonly available products (such as tissue paper and flour) that can help remove or adsorb the agent should be used if other decontaminants are not available.

PHARMACOLOGICAL TREATMENT WITH DIAZEPAM (VALIUM)

Diazepam, known more commonly as Valium, is an anticonvulsant of the benzodiazepine family that has been shown to control soman-induced convulsions in monkeys and convulsions induced by other ChE inhibitors in the rabbit. There have also been anecdotal reports of its effectiveness in controlling convulsions induced by organophosphate insecticides. In soman-poisoned rats, diazepam has been reported to decrease the frequency of convulsions and incidence of brain lesions (although, when given without atropine, it did not decrease mortality). During the Persian Gulf War, the U.S. military issued an autoinjector containing 10 mg of diazepam to all military personnel.

ATROPINE AND 2PAM CL

Under certain conditions, soldiers are routinely issued three MARK I kits. Each MARK I kit contains two autoinjectors: an AtroPen containing 2 mg of atropine in 0.7 milliliters (ml) of diluent and a ComboPen containing 600 mg of 2PAM Cl in 2 ml of diluent.

Atropine is the main nerve gas antidote. Atropine is a drug that blocks the effects of the excess acetylcholine at muscarinic acetylcholine receptor sites. In addition, 2-pyridine aldoxime methyl chloride (2PAM Cl, also called pralidoxime chloride) is an oxime that will remove the agent from acetylcholinesterase, thereby reactivating the enzyme after poisoning by some agents.

This ComboPen was not intended for self-use but rather for use by a buddy when a soldier exhibited severe effects from a nerve agent. (The buddy system was used because it is said that any soldier able to self-administer does not need it. But, based on interviews with experienced soldiers, we have been told they realize they may have to self-inject.)

Medics and unit lifesavers are also often issued additional diazepam autoinjectors and could administer two additional doses at 10-minute intervals to a convulsing casualty. The autoinjector is not only more convenient to use than the needle and syringe, but its use causes more rapid absorption of the drug. The AstroPen, on the other hand, sprays the liquid throughout the muscle as the needle goes in. The greater dispersion of the AtroPen deposit results in more rapid absorption.

Current policy states that diazepam is given following the third MARK I when three MARK I kits are given at one time. You can learn how to use MARK I kits by obtaining Meridian Auto-Injector Trainers available at www.domesticpreparedness.com. The contact is Meridian Medical Technologies, Inc., 10240 Old Columbia Road, Columbia, MD 21046. The phone number is (410) 309-6830 or toll free (800) 638-8093.

As a general rule, if a casualty is seen immediately after exposure from vapor only, the contents of one MARK I kit should be given if miosis is the only sign, the contents of two kits should be administered immediately if there is any dyspnea, and the contents of three kits should be given for severe dyspnea or any more severe signs or symptoms.

Source: The MARK I autoinjectors and their contents are manufactured by Survival Technology, Rockville, Maryland.

NUTRITIONAL PROTECTION

If you ride the New York or Washington, D.C. subway system, you may want to pretreat yourself or supplement your diet with huperzine A (HUP), an alkaloid isolated from the Chinese club moss *Huperzia serrata.*

Researchers reporting in 2001 in *Neurotoxicology* note that the herb may be useful against nerve gas poisoning.[1] Huperzine A is a reversible inhibitor of cholinesterases, which crosses the blood-brain barrier and shows high specificity for acetylcholinesterase (AChE) and a prolonged biological half-life.

In rats pretreated with 500 micrograms per kilogram body weight of HUP, the researchers observed that 93 percent of the animals survived and none of them had seizures. This dose of HUP reduced AChE inhibition to 54 percent. "HUP thus appears as a promising compound to protect subjects against organophosphorus intoxication," they said.

The ability of HUP to prevent seizures and subsequent hippocampal neuropathological changes induced by the organophosphate soman was studied in guinea pigs.[2] Pretreatment at 0.5 mg/kg, intraperitoneally, totally prevented seizures and ensured the survival of all animals for 24 hours after intoxication. Hippocampal tissue was then free of any neuronal damage. "In conclusion, HUP...protects against soman-induced convulsions and neuropathological changes in the hippocampus," said the researchers. "This efficacy seems to be related to a protection by HUP of both peripheral and central stores of AChE." These results are further supported by additional experimental work at the Israel Institute for Biological Research, Ness-Ziona.[3]

Keep in mind, however, that the lowest amount of HUP that was shown to be beneficial was 100 micrograms per kilogram of body weight, equivalent to approximately 7,000 mcg for humans—an amount that has not been confirmed safe for long-term use. That amount would also cost approximately $23.00 per day.

Still, if daily supplementation with a smaller amount offers even a few hours or minutes of added bodily resistance, such supplementation could well be worthwhile. We also know that HUP has beneficial effects on the memory at smaller dosages, which are thought to be safe. This material agent can be purchased at health food stores.

ANTIOXIDANT LEVELS CRITICAL

Recently, we have learned that our Gulf War veterans might well have been exposed to low levels of nerve gas, and that, while surviving these exposure, our men and women might suffer lasting effects. The Pentagon has identified about 130,000 troops it believes were exposed to low levels of sarin in 1991 when U.S. forces destroyed a weapons depot at Khamisiyah in southern Iraq. Some veterans believe other sarin exposures occurred.

This brings to mind why some are doing better than others. One reason might well be that some of our veterans had higher levels of circulating antioxidants, protecting their critical tissues, aiding the body in detoxification. For this reason, we urge you to maintain optimal antioxidant status. While a severe nerve gas attack might well overwhelm the body, in some cases your antioxidant status might offer just enough protection to survive. In addition, high levels of circulating antioxidants might reduce the severity of such exposures' debilitating and lingering after-effects.

"Low levels of sarin nerve gas affected behavior and organ functions in laboratory animals at least a month after exposure, suggests new research that may provide clues to the mysterious illnesses of Persian Gulf War veterans," notes a January 2003 report from Associated Press.

"In separate Army-sponsored studies, scientists observed behavioral problems, brain changes and immune system suppression in the animals many days after exposure to doses that caused no immediate effects, such as convulsions or pupil constriction.

"Both studies involved rodents, and 'that's a big leap to human beings,' said Melinda Roberson, a behavioral neuroscientist involved in a study still under way.

"Even so, the studies provide new information in an area where a lack of research has made it impossible to conclude whether Gulf veterans' illnesses are linked to low-level sarin gas exposure."

"They are pushing back the frontiers of biological effects of low levels of sarin. The evidence is building," said Dr. Francis O'Donnell, a medical consultant for the Defense Department who helps track Gulf War illness research.

Veterans of the 1991 war have suffered from various illnesses they believe linked to their service in the Gulf. Symptoms include chronic fatigue, diarrhea, migraines, dizziness, memory problems, loss of muscle control and loss of balance.

Most scientists have blamed stress. Some veterans attribute the health problems to toxic substances they encountered in the Gulf, including sarin, a toxic chemical weapon that is lethal at high levels. Others suggest it may be a combination of the factors.

Dr. Robert Haley, an epidemiologist at University of Texas Southwestern Medical Center at Dallas, has published almost two dozen studies suggesting that some Gulf War veterans' illnesses are linked to brain damage resulting from exposure to toxins such as sarin. The Pentagon criticized those studies, in part because veterans Haley studied were not downwind of Khamisiyah when the depot was destroyed. Haley said the new research gives "biological plausibility" to his suggestion of a link to sarin gas exposure.

The study on guinea pigs is under way at the Army Medical Research Institute for Chemical Defense at Aberdeen Proving Ground, Maryland. Its preliminary findings were presented in November at the Society for Neuroscience's annual meeting in Washington.

In that study, guinea pigs were injected with nerve gas five days a week for two weeks. Some were injected with 20 percent of the dose required to kill half the animals and others with 40 percent of that dose.

"Researcher Jim McDonough, a physiological psychologist, said that would be much higher than the level that the Pentagon says veterans were exposed to from the Khamisiyah depot destruction," notes the AP report. "Some veterans' groups question the accuracy of the Pentagon's exposure estimates, insisting they were much higher. Other researchers say there is no way to calculate the exposure levels for sure.

"Although veterans were not injected with sarin, McDonough said the biochemical effects on the brain are the same for either exposure method. He likened the exposures to nicotine's effects on the brain whether the nicotine is smoked, chewed or delivered through a skin patch.

"The exposed animals were examined after two hours, then at three days, 10 days, a month and 100 days. There were no changes in some physical signs the scientists monitored, such as weight gain and temperature. But researchers said they found significant increases in certain behaviors.

"For example, 100 days after exposure, animals in the 40 percent dose group spent significantly more time in the center of their activity chambers and traveled greater distances in the chambers, McDonough said. Guinea pigs in both dosage level groups also reared up on their hind legs significantly more often at 100 days.

"Separately, researchers at Lovelace Respiratory Research Institute in Albuquerque, known for its tobacco studies, exposed mice to low-level doses of sarin in a three-part Army-funded study. The study, begun in 1998, was finished last year.

"The mice inhaled sarin doses an hour a day for five days and an hour a day for 10 days. The levels were one-tenth and one-twentieth the concentrations required to kill a human. The mice were examined a day and a month after exposure."

"Researchers found that the exposures, particularly when combined with heat stress, caused both decreases and increases in the numbers of receptor sites in areas of the brain critical for cognition and memory, 'things that might be associated with Gulf War syndrome,'" said Rogene Henderson, Lovelace senior scientist.

Receptor sites are essentially docking stations for brain signals. In some cases the changes did not appear until a month after exposure.

Researchers found that the exposure also suppressed the immune system, the body's defense mechanism against infection and disease.

We think maintaining high antioxidant levels will help protect civilians and service personnel. In fact, it might be a great idea to make sure our service personnel are given antioxidant supplements with meals. The U.S. Army Medical Research and Materiel Command at Fort Detrick, Maryland, together with Meharry Medical College, Nashville, Tennesse, is researching antioxidant protectors given to animals dosed with mustard gas as a potential antidote. We think the same approach should be considered for nerve gas exposure. Their ability to support detoxification is well documented.

Guide to Antioxidants

Quite apart from threats of biological, chemical and nuclear terrorism, today, every one of us is under attack by a multitude of toxins. Interestingly, some of these chemical toxins, namely organophosphate pesticides, are considered to be less powerful "cousins" of nerve gas. Other toxins, such as low-level radiation, are less toxic "cousins" to what we might expect from use of radioactive "dirty" bombs. And, all of us are under attack, as well, from bacterial and viral pathogens that sometimes have been proven to be as deadly as the weaponized biological agents of terrorism.

Thus, in all of these instances, with both environmental exposures and potentially unique and devastating exposures to the weapons of terrorism, preservation of our health is at stake. Taking care to preserve your health in a toxic environment could also help to preserve your health in cases of biological, chemical and nuclear terrorism.

Health-conscious consumers can obtain much improved health—and preserve their health—by dramatically boosting circulating levels of antioxidants, a key aspect of detoxification, immune health and overall longevity.

Of course, no one element can be held responsible for protecting us from the myriad health challenges we face in today's complicated world, but antioxidants with their amazing ability to defuse toxins and free radicals come close.

Be sure to eat antioxidant-rich foods such as blueberries, raspberries, strawberries, apples, oranges, carrots, tomatoes, and all sorts of other fruits and vegetables, which help to counter free radical-related damage.

Also, be sure to supplement your diet with quality antioxidant formulas. Dietary and supplemental antioxidants are keys to prevention of premature aging, including reducing your risk of heart disease, cancer, diabetes, and almost all other age-related maladies. Here are some key antioxidants to seek:

Alpha-lipoic acid: Very potent and versatile, alpha-lipoic acid helps deactivate a wide array of fat- and water-soluble free radicals in many bodily systems. In particular, it may help protect the genetic material, DNA. It is also important because it works closely with vitamins C and E and some other antioxidants, "recycling" them and thus making them much more effective.

Bilberry: Especially helpful ophthalmologic disorders including myopia, diminished acuity, dark adaptation, macular degeneration, night blindness, diabetic retinopathy and cataracts, bilberry helps to prevent capillary permeability. Bilberry's anthocyanosides are thought to aid microvascular blood flow by intensifying arteriolar rhythmic diameter changes.

Bioflavonoids: Also known as vitamin P, these naturally occurring constituents of fruits are known individually as rutin, hesperidin, quercetin and naringin. Impressive clinical results have been obtained in the treatment of capillary permeability, easy bruising, hemorrhoids, and varicose veins.

Carotenoids: Including beta-carotene, lycopene, lutein, these important compounds have anticancer properties and are especially protective against cancer of the breast and prostate. Lycopene is thought to be the highest overall single oxygen-quenching carotenoid. Its activity is roughly double that of beta-carotene.

Coenzyme Q_{10} (CoQ_{10}): Not only a powerful antioxidant, CoQ_{10} is extremely beneficial for heart health and in cancer therapeutics. It also helps promote gum health and is considered to be a primary anti-aging supplement.

Ginkgo biloba: Not only a powerful antioxidant, ginkgo increases blood flow to the brain and throughout the body's network of blood vessels that supply blood and oxygen to the organ systems. Studies have confirmed that ginkgo increases blood flow to the retina, and can slow retinal deterioration. In clinical tests, ginkgo has improved hearing loss in the elderly. It also improves circulation in the extremities, relieving cold hands and feet, swelling in the limbs and chronic arterial blockage.

Glutathione: A small molecule found in almost every cell, the liver and kidneys contain high levels of glutathione, which is especially beneficial for detoxifying the body of cancer-causing chemicals, heavy metals, and toxic drug metabolites. Glutathione values decline with age and higher values in older people are seen to correlate with better health, underscoring the importance of this remarkable substance for maintaining a healthy, well-functioning body. Glutathione is produced in the body chiefly from three amino acids, glutamic acid, cysteine, and glycine. Also required is a support team of a combination of alpha-lipoic acid, riboflavin, zinc, and selenium.

Green tea: The polyphenols in this popular tea fight cancer, reduce blood pressure and prevent skin aging. Green tea is often used topically.

Milk thistle: A powerful antioxidant and liver protector, milk thistle is a mainstay of almost all antioxidant supplement formulas.

Pycnogenol®: This is a water extract from the bark of the French maritime pine grown in Europe's largest single forest, spread over the coastal region of southwest France. Pycnogenol is a powerful antioxidant that helps to relieve inflammation and pain, improves skin smoothness and elasticity, and reduces prostate inflammation and other inflammatory conditions, reduces diabetic retinopathy and neuropathy, improves circulation and enhances cell vitality.

Quercetin: Quercetin is a flavonol, a subclass of flavonoids, and is a potent antioxidant. Quercetin affects the formation of inflammatory mediators, which cause allergic reactions and asthma.

Rutin: Rich in quercetin, rutin staves off allergic reactions, helps to reduce blood clotting and, like all bioflavonoids, enhances the actions of vitamin C.

Selenium: This vital mineral, often deficient in the diet, is an important part of antioxidant enzymes that protect cells against the effects of free radicals that are produced during normal oxygen metabolism. Selenium is also essential for normal functioning of the immune system and thyroid gland. Plant foods are the major dietary sources of selenium in most countries throughout the world. Selenium also can be found in some meats and seafood. Some nuts, in particular Brazil nuts and walnuts, are also very good sources of selenium.

Superoxide dismutase (also known as SOD): One of the body's master antioxidants, this enzyme disarms members of the superoxide family of free radicals.

Turmeric: A widely used tropical herb and member of the ginger family, turmeric is rich in curcumin, which has powerful anticancer and anti-inflammatory properties.

Vitamin C: This vitamin works as an antioxidant in water environments in the body to "scavenge" peroxyl radicals before these destructive substances have a chance to damage cell membranes.

Vitamin E: A potent, fat soluble antioxidant, vitamin E is important in protecting cell membranes from oxidative damage.

Good antioxidant formulas can be found at your health food store. Be sure to seek a wide mix of antioxidants, as studies show antioxidants, incombination, tend to be synergistic.

CHAPTER THREE

Protecting Against Biological Weaons

During the Persian Gulf War (1990–1991), the United States and her coalition partners were faced with the credible and realistic threat that weapons of mass destruction, including biological agents, might be used by Iraq against allied forces. It is now known that Iraq had actually put offensive biological agents into several weapons systems for delivery. These revelations, combined with the fact that terrorist groups such as the Aum Shinrikyo in Japan have sought to produce biological agents, have catapulted the United States into an era where the use of biological warfare agents against our civilian population by terrorists is a possibility that we cannot ignore.

Defending against these agents requires us to understand how an adversary might use them. Biological agents must be considered in terms of an evolving world, where advances in modern technology and weapons delivery systems (e.g., long-range cruise missiles with multiple warheads) have overcome some of the earlier physical limitations.

A biological warfare agent need no longer be highly lethal to be effective, for incapacitation and confusion may be all the disruption necessary to cause the intended effects. Biological weapons may also be used in combination with other types of weapons or to add to the disruption produced by conventional weaponry. Finally, it would appear from the way conflict is evolving that nonconventional or terrorist use of biological agents is becoming more, rather than less, likely. The method for delivery of biological warfare agents may be as simple and inconspicuous as dropping an anthrax-containing letter into a post box to be delivered to a major media organization or congressional representative or, more ominously, attaching an off-the-shelf spray device to a car, truck, boat, or airplane—which appears harmless and normal to all who might observe the delivery vehicle.

Since initial symptoms resulting from a biological warfare agent may often be indistinguishable from those produced by endemic infections, a biological weapon may be capable of producing devastating health effects before the presence of the agent is even suspected. When one person falls victim, others may still be incubating the disease.

Biological warfare could be used against the United States in a theater of operations or against our civilian populations in any number of realistic scenarios. The medical consequences of such use are potentially catastrophic unless measures are taken to minimize the potential impact of biological warfare agents on our people. Proper planning for diseases that are likely to occur in the theater of operations is essential.

Many biological agents, including bacteria, viruses, and toxins, can be used as biological weapons.

POSSIBLE BIOLOGICAL WARFARE AGENTS

Bacteria

Bacillus anthracis (anthrax)
Yersinia pestis (plague)
Francisella tularensis (tularemia)
Brucella species (brucellosis)
Coxiella burnetii (Q fever)

Viruses

Variola virus (smallpox)
Equine encephalitis viruses (viral equine encephalitides)
Arenaviruses, bunyaviruses, filoviruses, flaviviruses (hemorrhagic fevers)

Toxins

Staphylococcal enterotoxin B
Ricin
Botulinum toxins
Trichothecene mycotoxins
Saxitoxin

HOW BIOLOGICAL AGENTS WORK

Biological warfare agents are likely to be selected for their ability to either incapacitate or kill the human targets of the attack. A biological warfare agent does not necessarily have to be lethal to be useful as a military weapon. An agent such as Venezuelan equine encephalitis (VEE) virus could terrorize entire populations by simply incapacitating large numbers of persons.

If one of an adversary's aims is to overload our field medical care systems, an incapacitating agent such as VEE virus might be chosen preferentially to a lethal biological agent. If death is desired, agents such as *Bacillus anthracis* (anthrax), the viruses that cause Ebola hemorrhagic fever, Marburg disease, and Crimean Congo hemorrhagic fever, or the plague bacillus, *Yersinia pestis*, might be used.

Inhalational anthrax, pneumonic plague, and certain viral hemorrhagic fevers have high fatality rates once infection is established in nonimmune hosts. Viruses may be particularly attractive as biological warfare agents because specific treatments are not available for many of them. Agents that require low doses to produce their intended effects—whether lethality, incapacitation, or intoxication—would, for logistical and tactical reasons, have greater utility as biological weapons.

Although, in general, a shorter incubation time to onset of deleterious effects is desirable, this characteristic would vary according to the aims of the aggressor. Very short incubation periods might be more useful in a tactical setting, whereas longer incubation times would work to the advantage of the terrorist, assassin, or special forces unit in order to enable them to escape prior to the onset of the effects of the attack.

Very few biological agents are immediately lethal. Some of the most toxic toxins, such as saxitoxin, are available only in small quantities, but an adversary could use these as assassination or antipersonnel weapons. Certain penetrating devices designed to be used with such toxins, such as flechettes, have been developed in the past.

Biowarfare agents might be released by an aggressor against our forces or against civilian populations by means of sprays, explosive devices, and contamination of food and water. Most commonly, delivery methods use aerosolized agents.

There are four basic scenarios for criminal or terrorist attacks with biological agents. The following examples demonstrate that terrorist acts have already occurred using chemical agents:

1. Product tampering (e.g., the Tylenol tampering cases of the 1980s).
2. Attacks on specific ethnic population groups within a country who are perceived to be in opposition to terrorist goals.
3. Sabotage of specific food groups or industries, such as contamination of an imported food product with a toxin, pathogenic bacteria, or poison (e.g., the lacing with cyanide of Chilean grapes in March 1989).
4. Attacks directed at one of a country's institutions, agencies, or departments, such as the military, a stock market, or a major communications center.

ANTHRAX

During the latter half of the 19th century, a previously unrecognized form of anthrax appeared for the first time, namely, inhalational anthrax. This occurred among woolsorters in England, due to the generation of infectious aerosols of anthrax spores under industrial conditions, from the processing of contaminated goat hair and alpaca wool. It probably represents the first described occupational respiratory infectious disease.

Owing to the infectiousness of anthrax spores by the respiratory route and the high mortality of inhalational anthrax, the military's concern with anthrax is with its potential use as a biological weapon. This concern was heightened by the revelation that the largest epidemic of inhalational anthrax in this century, in Sverdlovsk, Russia, in 1979, occurred after anthrax spores were released from a military research facility located upwind from where the cases occurred. Cases were also reported in animals located more than 50 kilometers from the site.

Anthrax, a zoonotic disease caused by *Bacillus anthracis*, occurs in domesticated and wild animals—primarily herbivores, including goats, sheep, cattle, horses, and swine. Humans usually become infected by contact with infected animals or contaminated animal products. Infection occurs most commonly via the cutaneous route and only very rarely via the respiratory or gastrointestinal routes. Anthrax has a long association with human history.

The fifth and sixth plagues described in Exodus may have been anthrax in domesticated animals followed by cutaneous anthrax in humans. The disease that Virgil described in his *Georgics* is clearly anthrax in domestic and wild animals. And during the 16th to the 18th centuries in Europe, anthrax was an economically important agricultural disease.

Anthrax was intimately associated with the origins of microbiology and immunology, being the first disease for which a microbial origin was definitively established, in 1876, by Robert Koch.

Anthrax occurs worldwide. The organism exists in the soil as a spore. The question remains unsettled as to whether its persistence in the soil is due to significant multiplication of the organism in the soil or if it is due solely to cycles of bacterial amplification in infected animals whose carcasses then contaminate the soil.

Inhalational anthrax begins after an incubation period of one to six days with nonspecific symptoms of malaise, fatigue, myalgia, and fever. There may be an associated nonproductive cough and mild chest discomfort. These symptoms usually persist for two or three days, and in some cases there may be a short period of improvement. This is followed by the sudden onset of increasing respiratory distress with dyspnea, stridor (a harsh, vibrating sound heard during respiration in cases of obstruction of the air passages), cyanosis, increased chest pain, and diaphoresis. There may be associated edema of the chest and neck. Chest X-ray examination usually shows the characteristic widening of the mediastinum and, often, pleural effusions. Pneumonia has not been a consistent finding but can occur in some patients.

The antibiotic of choice for treating anthrax is ciprofloxcin (Cipro).

PLAGUE

Plague is a zoonotic infection caused by *Yersinia pestis*, a Gram-negative bacillus, which has been the cause of three great pandemics of human disease in the common era—in the 6th, 14th, and 20th centuries.

The naturally occurring disease in humans is transmitted from rodents and is characterized by the abrupt onset of high fever, painful local lymphadenopathy draining the exposure site (i.e., a *bubo*, the inflammatory swelling of one or more lymph nodes, usually in the groin; the confluent mass of nodes, if untreated, may suppurate and drain pus), and bacteremia. Septicemic plague can sometimes ensue from untreated bubonic plague or, *de novo*, after a flea bite. Patients with the bubonic form of the disease may develop secondary pneumonic plague (also called plague pneumonia). This complication can lead to human-to-human spread by the respiratory route and cause primary pneumonic plague, the most severe and frequently fatal form of the disease.

During the last four millennia, plague has played a role in many military campaigns. During the Vietnam War, plague was endemic among the native population, but U.S. soldiers escaped relatively unaffected. This excellent protection of troops was largely due to our understanding of the rodent reservoirs and flea vectors of disease, the pathophysiology of the various clinical forms of plague, the widespread use throughout the war of a plague vaccine, and prompt treatment of plague victims with effective antibiotics.

Mortality from endemic plague continues at low rates throughout the world despite the availability of effective antibiotics. People continue to die of plague, not because the bacilli have become resistant but, most often, because physicians do not include plague in their differential diagnosis (in the United States) or because treatment is absent or delayed (in underdeveloped countries).

The United States military's concern with plague is both as an endemic disease and as a biological warfare threat. A better understanding of the preventive medicine aspects of the disease will aid in the prompt diagnosis and effective treatment necessary to survive an enemy attack of plague.

All patients with plague should be isolated for the first 48 hours after the initiation of treatment. Special care must be taken in handling blood and bubo discharge. If pneumonic plague is present, then strict, rigidly enforced respiratory isolation procedures must be followed, including the use of gowns, gloves, and eye protection. Patients with pneumonia must be isolated until they have completed at least four days of antibiotic therapy. If patients have no pneumonia or draining lesions at 48 hours, they may be taken out of strict isolation.

Since 1948, streptomycin has remained the treatment of choice for bubonic, septicemic, and pneumonic plague. It should be given intramuscularly in a dose of 30 milligrams per kilogram body weight per day (mg/kg/d) in two divided doses. In cases of suspected meningitis or in patients who are hemodynamically unstable, intravenous chloramphenicol (50–75 mg/kg/d in four divided doses) should be added. Gentamicin has had much less clinical usage but can be used as an alternative.

Streptomycin should be administered alone or together with chloramphenicol. Treatment should be continued for a minimum of 10 days or three to four days after clinical recovery. If clinically indicated, oral tetracycline can be used to complete a 10-day course of treatment after at least five days of systemic therapy. In patients with very mild bubonic plague who are not septic, tetracycline can be used orally at a dose of two grams per day (g/d) in four divided doses for 10 days. Doxycycline should be an acceptable alternative, although there are no published data on its efficacy in humans. Doxycycline, ofloxacin, and ceftriaxone have all been shown to be effective in experimental animal models of septicemic plague.

In pregnant women, streptomycin or gentamicin should be used unless chloramphenicol is specifically indicated. Streptomycin is also the treatment of choice in newborns.

If treated with antibiotics, buboes typically recede in 10 to 14 days and do not require drainage.

Patients are unlikely to survive primary pneumonic plague if antibiotic therapy is not initiated within 18 hours of the onset of symptoms. Without treatment, mortality is 60 percent for bubonic plague and 100 percent for the pneumonic and septicemic forms. It might be worthwhile, therefore, to have these antibiotics on hand in your medicine cabinet for such emergencies.

TULAREMIA

F. tularensis has been considered an important biological warfare threat because of its very high infectivity after aerosolization. Tularemia is a zoonosis caused by the Gram-negative, facultative intracellular bacterium, *Francisella tularensis.* The disease is characterized by fever, localized skin or mucous membrane ulceration, regional lymphadenopathy, and, occasionally, pneumonia.

In 1911, G. W. McCoy discovered the disease in Tulare County, California, as a cause of a plaguelike illness in ground squirrels. An organism was isolated and named *Bacterium tularense.*

Tularemia can be divided into the ulceroglandular (75 percent of patients) and the typhoidal (25 percent of patients) forms, based on the clinical signs. Patients with ulceroglandular tularemia have lesions on the skin or mucous membranes (including the conjunctiva), lymph nodes larger than one centimeter in diameter, or both. Patients with typhoidal tularemia, on the other hand, have lymph nodes smaller than one cm in diameter and no skin or mucous membrane lesions.

After an incubation period of three to six days, patients with the ulceroglandular form of the disease develop a constellation of symptoms consisting of fever (85%), chills (52%), headache (45%), cough (38%), and myalgias (31%). Patients may also complain of chest pain, vomiting, arthralgia, sore throat, abdominal pain, diarrhea, dysuria, back pain, or stiff neck.

A cutaneous ulcer occurs in approximately 60 percent of patients and is the most common sign of tularemia. Ulcers are generally single lesions of 0.4 to 3.0 cm in diameter, with heaped-up edges.

Lesions associated with infection acquired from mammalian vectors are usually located on the upper extremities, whereas lesions associated with infection acquired from arthropod vectors are usually located on the lower extremities. Ulcerative lesions are almost always accompanied by enlarged lymph glands and accumulation of lymph fluid.

Enlarged lymph nodes are seen in approximately 85% of patients, and may be the initial, or the only, sign of infection. Nodes are usually tender and 0.5 to 10 cm in diameter (mean 2.0 cm).

Patients with tularemia who do not receive appropriate antibiotic treatment may have a prolonged illness characterized by malaise, weakness, weight loss, and other symptoms that last for months. With appropriate treatment, tularemia has an overall mortality of approximately 1 to 2.5 percent.

Streptomycin is the drug of choice for the treatment of tularemia. The drug is bactericidal, and patients treated with streptomycin usually respond within 48 hours of its administration. Relapses are uncommon and resistance has not been reported.

Other aminoglycosides, such as gentamicin, have been used with some success and are probably reasonable alternatives. Bacteriostatic drugs, such as chloramphenicol and tetracycline, are often efficacious but relapses occur if the drug is given too early in the course of the disease or if is not continued long enough.

BRUCELLOSIS

The ease of transmission by aerosol suggests that *Brucella* organisms might be a candidate for use as a biological warfare agent. Indeed, the United States began development of B suis as a biological weapon in 1942. The agent was formulated to maintain long-term viability, placed into bombs, and tested in field trials during 1944–1945 using animal targets. By 1967, the United States terminated its offensive program for development and deployment of *Brucella* as a biological weapon. Although the munitions developed were never used in combat, the studies reinforced the concern that *Brucella* organisms might be used against U.S. troops as a biological warfare agent.

Brucellae are small, nonmotile, nonsporulating, nontoxigenic, nonfermenting, aerobic, Gram-negative coccobacilli that may, based on DNA homology, represent a single species.

Clinical manifestations of brucellosis are diverse and the course of the disease is variable. Patients with brucellosis may have with an acute, systemic febrile illness; an insidious chronic infection; or a localized inflammatory process. Disease may be abrupt or insidious in onset, with an incubation period of three days to several weeks. Patients usually complain of nonspecific symptoms such as fever, sweats, fatigue, anorexia, and muscle or joint aches. Neuropsychiatric symptoms, notably depression, headache, and irritability, occur frequently.

In addition, focal infection of bone, joints, or genitourinary tract may cause local pain. Cough, pleuritic chest pain, and dyspepsia may also be noted. Symptoms of patients infected by aerosol are indistinguishable from those of patients infected by other routes.

Chronically infected patients frequently lose weight. Symptoms often last for three to six months and occasionally for a year or more. Physical examination is usually normal, although hepatomegaly, splenomegaly, or lymphadenopathy may occur. Brucellosis does not usually cause leukocytosis, and some patients may be moderately neutropenic.

Brucellae are sensitive to a number of oral antibiotics and to aminoglycosides. Therapy with a single drug has resulted in a high relapse rate, so combined regimens should be used whenever possible.

A six-week regimen of doxycycline 200 mg/d administered orally, with the addition of streptomycin 1 g/d administered intramuscularly for the first 2 to 3 weeks is effective therapy for adults with most forms of brucellosis.

Several studies suggest that treatment with a combination of streptomycin and doxycycline may result in less frequent relapse than treatment with the combination of rifampin and doxycycline. The Joint Food and Agriculture Organization–World Health Organization Expert Committee recommends treatment of pregnant women with rifampin.

In the event of a biological attack, the standard gas mask should adequately protect personnel from airborne brucellae since the organisms are probably unable to penetrate intact skin. After personnel have been evacuated from the attack area, clothing, skin, and other surfaces can be decontaminated with standard disinfectants to minimize risk of infection by accidental ingestion, or by conjunctival inoculation of viable organisms. There is no commercially available vaccine for humans.

Q FEVER

Q fever is a zoonotic disease caused by *Coxiella burnetii*, a rickettsia-like organism of low virulence but remarkable infectivity. A single organism may initiate infection. In addition, despite the fact that *C. burnetii* is unable to grow or replicate outside host cells, there is a sporelike form of the organism that is extremely resistant to heat, pressure, desiccation, and many standard antiseptic compounds; this allows *C. burnetii* to persist in the environment for long periods (weeks or months) under harsh conditions. This persistence, coupled with a primary mode of transmission by inhalation of infected aerosols, allows for the development of acute infection following only indirect exposure to an infected source.

In contrast to this high degree of inherent resilience and transmissibility, the acute clinical disease associated with Q fever infection is usually a benign, although a temporarily incapacitating, illness in humans. Even without treatment, the vast majority of patients recover. Chronic disease as a result of Q fever is rare, although it is frequently fatal. The primary reservoir for natural human infection is livestock, particularly parturient females, and the distribution is worldwide.

The potential of *C. burnetii* as a biological warfare threat is directly related to its infectivity. It has been estimated that 50 kilograms of dried, powdered *C. burnetii* would produce casualties at a rate equal to that of similar amounts of anthrax or tularemia organisms.

Human infection with *C. burnetii* is usually the result of inhalation of infected aerosols. Following this, the organisms are phagocytized by host cells, predominately unstimulated macrophages. This uptake of *C. burnetii* by host phagocytic cells is not energy dependent but is probably the result of contact by the pathogen with an existing receptor. After phagocytosis by host cells, conditions within the phagolysosome trigger growth and multiplication of *C. burnetii*, with little initial damage to the host cell. Eventually the cytoplasm becomes engorged with *C. burnetii* organisms and lysis of the host cell occurs. Dissemination of the pathogen occurs as a result of circulation of organisms free in the plasma, on the surface of cells, and carried by circulating macrophages.

Humans are the only host susceptible to infection by *C. burnetii* and that commonly develops an illness as a result of the infection. The incubation period varies from 10 to 40 days, with the duration of the incubation period being inversely correlated with the magnitude of the inoculum.

When symptomatic, the onset of Q fever may be abrupt or insidious, with fever, chills (including frank rigors), and headache being the most common signs and symptoms. The headache is usually described as severe, throbbing, and frontal or retroorbital in location. Diaphoresis, malaise, fatigue, and anorexia are also very common.

Tetracyclines have been the mainstay of therapy since the 1950s. When initiated within the first few days of illness, treatment with a tetracycline shortens the course of the disease. Attempted prophylaxis with a tetracycline (20 grams of oxytetracycline administered over five to six days), however, has produced mixed results.

Initiation of the antibiotic early in the incubation period (24 hours after exposure) merely prolonged the incubation period, while initiation of therapy late in the incubation period prevented the development of disease.

Macrolide antibiotics, such as erythromycin, are also effective for the treatment of acute Q fever. A new macrolide, azithromycin, has also demonstrated efficacy in a few cases, but experience is very limited. At least two years of therapy are required, usually with a tetracycline combined with rifampin or a quinolone, although trimethoprim sulfamethoxazole has also been used. Quinolones alone or in combination have also been effective. Most recently, the addition of hydroxychloroquine to tetracycline has shown promising results both *in vitro* and in a small number of patients.

SMALLPOX

The poxviruses (of the family *Poxviridae*) are a family of large, enveloped deoxyribonucleic acid (DNA) viruses. The most notorious poxvirus is variola, the causative agent of smallpox. Smallpox was an important cause of morbidity and mortality in the developing world until recent times.

Since the host range of the variola virus is confined to humans, aggressive case identification and contact vaccination were ultimately successful in controlling the disease. The last occurrence of endemic smallpox was in Somalia in 1977, and the last human cases were laboratory-acquired infections in 1978. By 1980, the World Health Organization (WHO) General Assembly ratified the declaration of success made by the Global Commission for the Certification of Smallpox Eradication.

The concept of using variola virus in warfare is an old one. British colonial commanders considered distributing blankets from smallpox victims among Native Americans as a biological weapon. During the American Civil War, allegations were made about the use of smallpox as a biological weapon, although there subsequently proved to be no definite evidence for such. In the years leading up to and during World War II, the Japanese military explored weaponization of smallpox during the operations of Unit 731 in Mongolia and China.

Nevertheless, the actual potential of variola virus as a biological weapon remains controversial. Given the ease of administration and the availability of the vaccinia virus as a vaccine against smallpox, some have argued that smallpox would have limited biological warfare potential.

The discontinuation of routine vaccination has rendered civilian and military populations more susceptible to a disease that is not only infectious by aerosol but also infamous for its devastating morbidity and mortality. WHO voiced concerns that smallpox "can easily be produced in large quantities in the laboratory and... freeze-dried and its virulence thus preserved for months or years."

Since 1983, there have existed two WHO-approved and inspected repositories of variola virus: the CDC in the United States and Vector Laboratories in Russia. WHO continues to debate whether, given the completion of sequencing of several reference strains, all stocks of variola virus should be destroyed. Proponents of retaining these smallpox stocks argue that military or terrorist use of variola virus as a weapon would readily be countered by rigorous case contact evaluation and vaccination.

Variola virus is highly stable and retains its infectivity for long periods outside the host. It is infectious by aerosol, but natural airborne spreading of it by other than close contacts is controversial.

Patients with smallpox were infectious from the time of onset of their eruptive exanthem, most commonly from days three through six after onset of fever. Infectivity was markedly enhanced if the patient manifested a cough. Indirect transmission via contaminated bedding or other fomites was infrequent. Some close contacts harbored virus in their throats without developing disease, and hence might have served as a means of secondary transmission. The incubation period of smallpox averages 12 days, and contacts are quarantined for a minimum of 16 to 17 days following exposure.

Patients should be isolated and considered infectious until all scabs separate. For the past century, two distinct types of smallpox have been recognized. Variola major, the prototypical disease, was prevalent in Asia and parts of Africa. Variola minor, or alastrim, was distinguished by milder systemic toxicity and more diminutive pox lesions. Variola minor was found in Africa, South America, and Europe before the eradication of endemic disease and caused one percent mortality in unvaccinated victims.

Early attempts to control smallpox included inoculation with material from smallpox lesions. This practice, known as variolization, caused severe cases of smallpox in about 1 in 200 inoculations.

In 1796, Jenner noted that milkmaids were free of the facial scars that marked most of the population during the smallpox epidemics of that time. The observation that they "cannot take smallpox" was attributed to the localized pox lesions that they developed on their hands. Jenner reasoned that infectious material (which he dubbed a "virus") from cowpox lesions provided protection from smallpox, and he used it to vaccinate an 8-year-old boy. The boy later resisted variolation, demonstrating that an animal poxvirus that is not virulent for humans could be used as a potent vaccine against smallpox.

Evidence indicates that vaccinia-immune globulin (VIG) is of value in postexposure prophylaxis of smallpox when given (a) within the first week following exposure and (b) concurrently with vaccination. However, the prophylactic use of VIG should be carefully weighed vis-à-vis the risk of attenuating the immune response to booster vaccination.

VIG is available in the United States from the Drug Service of the CDC. The U.S. Army maintains a supply for its own use. The dose for prophylaxis or treatment is 0.6 milliliter per kilogram (mL/kg), administered intramuscularly.

Administration immediately after or within the first 24 hours of exposure would provide the highest level of protection, especially in unvaccinated persons. VIG is prepared from the plasma of repeatedly vaccinated persons.

THE SMALLPOX VACCINE

After the events of September and October 2001, the U.S. government took further actions to improve its level of preparedness against terrorism. One of many such measures—designed specifically to prepare for an intentional release of the smallpox virus—included ordering production of enough smallpox vaccine to immunize the American public in the event of a smallpox outbreak. Right now, the U.S. government has access to enough smallpox vaccine to effectively respond to a smallpox outbreak in the United States.

The smallpox vaccine helps the body develop immunity to smallpox. The vaccine is made from a virus called *vaccinia* which is a "pox"-type virus related to smallpox. The smallpox vaccine contains the "live" vaccinia virus—not dead virus like many other vaccines. For that reason, the vaccination site must be cared for carefully to prevent the virus from spreading. Also, the vaccine can have side effects (see below). The vaccine does not contain the smallpox virus and cannot give you smallpox.

Currently, the United States has a big enough stockpile of smallpox vaccine to vaccinate everyone in the country who might need it in the event of an emergency. Production of new vaccine is underway.

Historically, the vaccine has been effective in

preventing smallpox infection in 95 percent of those vaccinated. In addition, the vaccine was proven to prevent or substantially lessen infection when given within a few days of exposure. It is important to note, however, that at the time when the smallpox vaccine was used to eradicate the disease, testing was not as advanced or precise as it is today, so there may still be things to learn about the vaccine and its effectiveness and length of protection.

Receiving the Vaccine

The smallpox vaccine is not given with a hypodermic needle. It is not a shot as most people have experienced. The vaccine is given using a bifurcated (two-pronged) needle that is dipped into the vaccine solution. When removed, the needle retains a droplet of the vaccine. The needle is used to prick the skin a number of times in a few seconds. The pricking is not deep, but it will cause a sore spot and one or two droplets of blood to form. The vaccine usually is given in the upper arm.

If the vaccination is successful, a red and itchy bump develops at the vaccine site in three or four days. In the first week, the bump becomes a large blister, fills with pus, and begins to drain. During the second week, the blister begins to dry up and a scab forms. The scab falls off in the third week, leaving a small scar. People who are being vaccinated for the first time have a stronger reaction than those who are being revaccinated.

Post-vaccination Care

After vaccination, it is important to follow care instructions for the site of the vaccine. Because the virus is live, it can spread to other parts of the body, or to other people. The vaccinia virus (the live virus in the smallpox vaccine) may cause rash, fever, and head and body aches. In certain groups of people (see below), complications from the vaccinia virus can be severe.

Benefit of Vaccine Following Exposure

Vaccination within three days of exposure will prevent or significantly lessen the severity of smallpox symptoms in the vast majority of people. Vaccination four to seven days after exposure likely offers some protection from disease or may modify the severity of disease.

Smallpox Vaccine Safety

The smallpox vaccine is the best protection you can get if you are exposed to the smallpox virus. Anyone directly exposed to smallpox, regardless of health status, would be offered the smallpox vaccine because the risks associated with smallpox disease are far greater than those posed by the vaccine.

There are side effects and risks associated with the smallpox vaccine. Most people experience normal, usually mild reactions that include a sore arm, fever, and body aches. However, other people experience reactions ranging from serious to life threatening. People most likely to have serious side effects are: people who have had, even once, skin conditions (especially eczema or atopic dermatitis) and people with weakened immune systems, such as those who have received a transplant, are HIV positive, are receiving treatment for cancer, or are currently taking medications (like steroids) that suppress the immune system. In addition, pregnant women should not get the vaccine because of the risk it poses to the fetus. Women who are breastfeeding should not get the vaccine. Children younger than 12 months of age should not get the vaccine. Also, the Advisory Committee on Immunization Practices (ACIP) advises against non-emergency use of smallpox vaccine in children younger than 18 years of age. In addition, those allergic to the vaccine or any of its components should not receive the vaccine.

In the past, about 1,000 people for every one million people vaccinated for the first time experienced reactions that, while not life-threatening, were serious. These reactions included a toxic or allergic reaction at the site of the vaccination (erythema multiforme), spread of the vaccinia virus to other parts of the body and to other individuals (inadvertent inoculation), and spread of the vaccinia virus to other parts of the body through the blood (generalized vaccinia). These types of reactions may require medical attention. In the past, between 14 and 52 people out of every one million people vaccinated for the first time experienced potentially life-threatening reactions to the vaccine. Based on past experience, it is estimated that one or two people in one million who receive the vaccine may die as a result. Careful screening of potential vaccine recipients is essential to ensure that those at increased risk do not receive the vaccine.

Some people are at greater risk for serious side effects from the smallpox vaccine. Individuals who have any of the following conditions, or live with someone who does, should NOT get the smallpox vaccine unless they have been exposed to the smallpox virus:

- Eczema or atopic dermatitis. (This is true even if the condition is not currently active, mild or experienced as a child.)
- Skin conditions such as burns, chickenpox, shingles, impetigo, herpes, severe acne, or psoriasis. (People with any of these conditions should not get the vaccine until they have completely healed.)
- Weakened immune system. (Cancer treatment,

an organ transplant, HIV, some severe autoimmune disorders and medications to treat autoimmune disorders, and other illnesses can weaken the immune system.)

- Pregnancy or plans to become pregnant within one month of vaccination.

In addition, individuals should not get the smallpox vaccine if they:

- Are allergic to the vaccine or any of its ingredients.
- Are younger than 12 months of age. However, the Advisory Committee on Immunization Practices (ACIP) advises against non-emergency use of smallpox vaccine in children younger than 18 years of age. In addition, the vaccine manufacturer's package insert states that the vaccine is not recommended for use in geriatric populations in non-emergency situations. The term geriatric generally applies to those age 65 and above.
- Have a moderate or severe short-term illness. (These people should wait until they are completely recovered to get the vaccine.)
- Are currently breastfeeding.
- Are using steroid drops in their eyes. (These people should wait until they are no longer using the medication to get the vaccine.)

Again, people who have been directly exposed to the smallpox virus should get the

vaccine, regardless of their health status. Don't Hesitate!

If offered the smallpox vaccine, individuals should tell their immunization provider if they have any of the above conditions, or even if they suspect they might.

VIRAL ENCEPHALITIDES

During the 1930s, three distinct but antigenically related viruses were recovered from moribund horses and were shown to be previously unrecognized agents of severe equine encephalitis. Western equine encephalitis (WEE) virus was isolated in the San Joaquin Valley in California in 1930, eastern equine encephalitis (EEE) virus in Virginia and New Jersey in 1933, and Venezuelan equine encephalitis (VEE) virus in the Guajira peninsula of Venezuela in 1938.

By 1938, it was clear that EEE and WEE viruses were also natural causes of encephalitis in humans, and naturally acquired human infections with VEE virus were documented in Colombia in 1952 in association with an equine epizootic.

Although these viruses cause similar clinical syndromes in horses, the consequences of the infections they cause in humans differ. EEE is the most severe of the arboviral encephalitides, with case fatality rates of 50% to 70% and with neurological sequelae common in survivors. WEE virus appears to be less neuroinvasive but has a pathology similar to that of EEE in patients with encephalitis. In contrast, severe encephalitis is rare in humans infected with VEE virus—except in children. In adults, the usual VEE syndrome is an acute, febrile, incapacitating disease with prolonged convalescence.

The three viruses under discussion in this section are all members of the alphavirus genus of the family *Togaviridae*. As with all the alphavirus group, VEE, EEE, and WEE are transmitted in nature by mosquitoes and are maintained in cycles with various vertebrate hosts. Thus, the natural epidemiology of these viruses is controlled by environmental factors that affect the relevant mosquito and reservoir host populations and their interactions. Of the 28 viruses currently classified within this group, VEE, EEE, and WEE are the only viruses regularly associated with encephalitis. Although these encephalitic strains are restricted to the Americas, as a group, alphaviruses have worldwide distribution and include other epidemic human pathogens such as chikungunya virus (Asia and Africa), Mayaro virus (South America), O'nyongnyong virus (Africa), Ross River virus (Australia), and Sindbis virus (Africa, Europe, and Asia). These viruses cause an acute febrile syndrome often associated with debilitating polyarthritic syndromes.

Although natural infections with the encephalitic alphaviruses are acquired by mosquito bite, the viruses are also highly infectious by aerosol. VEE virus has caused more laboratory-acquired disease than any other arbovirus. Since its initial isolation, at least 150 laboratory infections that have resulted in disease have been reported; most were known or thought to be aerosol infections.

Before vaccines were developed, most laboratories working with VEE virus reported disease among their personnel. In one incident reported in 1959 at the Ivanovskii Institute in Moscow, USSR, at least 20 individuals developed disease, most within 28 to 33 hours, after an accident in which a small number of vials containing a minute amount of lyophilized virus were dropped and broken in a stairwell.

Perhaps as a consequence of their adaptation to dissimilar hosts in nature, the alphaviruses replicate readily, and generally to very high titers, in a wide range of cell types and culture conditions *in vitro*. Virus titers of 1 billion infectious units per milliliter are not unusual, and the viruses are stable in storage and in a variety of laboratory procedures.

Because of the relative ease with which these viruses can be manipulated in the laboratory, they have long served as model systems by which to study various aspects of virus replication, pathogenesis, induction of immune responses, and virus–vector relationships. As a result, the alpha viruses are well described and their characteristics well defined.

Therefore, the collective *in vitro* and *in vivo* characteristics of alphaviruses, especially the equine encephalomyelitis viruses, lend themselves very well to weaponization. This fact was recognized by the designers of offensive biological warfare programs that were initiated before or during World War II.

Although other encephalitic viruses could be considered as potential weapons (e.g., the tickborne encephalitis viruses), few possess as many of the required characteristics for strategic or tactical weapons development as the alphaviruses:

- These viruses can be produced in large amounts in inexpensive and unsophisticated systems.
- They are relatively stable and highly infectious for humans as aerosols.
- Strains are available that produce either incapacitating or lethal infections.
- The existence of multiple serotypes of VEE and EEE viruses, as well as the inherent difficulties of inducing efficient mucosal immunity, confound defensive vaccine development.

The equine encephalomyelitis viruses remain as highly credible threats today, and intentional release as a small particle aerosol from a single airplane could be expected to infect a high percentage of individuals within an area of at least 10,000 square kilometers. As a further complication, these viruses are readily amenable to genetic manipulation by modern recombinant deoxyribonucleic acid (DNA) technology.

This capability is being used to develop safer and more effective vaccines, but, in theory, could also be used to increase the weaponization potential of these viruses.

VIRAL HEMORRHAGIC FEVERS (VHFs)

The VHF agents are all highly infectious via the aerosol route, and most are quite stable as respirable aerosols (VHFs). This means that they satisfy at least one criterion for being weaponized, and some clearly have the potential to be biological warfare threats. Most of these agents replicate in cell culture to concentrations sufficiently high to produce a small terrorist weapon, one suitable for introducing lethal doses of virus into the air intake of an airplane or office building. Some replicate to even higher concentrations, with obvious potential ramifications.

Since the VHF agents cause serious diseases with high morbidity and mortality, their existence as endemic disease threats and as potential biological warfare weapons suggests a formidable public health concern.

The concept of a viral hemorrhagic fever (VHF) syndrome is useful in clinical medicine. The VHF syndrome can be described as an acute febrile illness characterized by malaise, prostration, generalized signs of increased vascular permeability, and abnormalities of circulatory regulation. Bleeding manifestations often occur, especially in the more severely ill patients, but this does not result in a life-threatening loss of blood volume. Rather, these signs are the result of damage to the vascular endothelium and are an index of how severe the disease is in specific target organs.

The viral agents that cause VHFs are taxonomically diverse; they are all ribonucleic acid (RNA) viruses and are transmitted to humans through contact with infected animal reservoirs or arthropod vectors. They are all natural infectious disease threats although their geographical ranges may be tightly circumscribed. The recent advent of jet travel coupled with human demographics increases the likelihood of cross-continental exposure.

These viruses tend to be stable and highly infectious as fine particle aerosols. These characteristics have great significance in the natural transmission cycle for arenaviruses and bunyaviruses (from rodents to man) and also make nosocomial (hospital) transmission a concern. As a group, the viruses are also linked to the ecology of their vectors or reservoirs, whether rodents or arthropods.

NEUROTOXINS

Saxitoxin

Some neurotoxins, such as saxitoxin and tetrodotoxin, can kill an individual very quickly after inhalation of a lethal dose (within minutes). These toxins act by blocking nerve conduction directly and cause death by paralyzing muscles of respiration. Yet, at just less than a lethal dose, the exposed individual may not even feel ill or may only feel dizzy. Because of the rapid onset of signs after inhalation, prophylaxis (either immunization or pretreatment) would be required to protect civilians from these two rapidly acting neurotoxins. Unprotected persons who inhale a lethal dose would probably die before they could be helped, unless they could be intubated and artificially ventilated immediately. Although the mechanism of death after inhalation of saxitoxin is believed to be the same as when the toxin is administered intravenously, it is more toxic if inhaled.

Botulinum

Other neurotoxins, such as the botulinum toxins, must enter nerve terminals before they can block the release of neurotransmitters, which normally cause muscle contraction. These largeprotein neurotoxins generally kill by relatively slow onset respiratory failure (within hours to days). The intoxicated individual may not show signs of disease for 24 to 72 hours. The toxin blocks biochemical action in the nerves that activate the muscles necessary for respiration, leading to suffocation. Intoxications such as this can be treated with antitoxin injected hours after exposure to a lethal dose of toxin (less than 24 hours in monkeys and probably also in humans) and illness and death can still be prevented. Although the mechanisms of toxicity of the botulinum toxins appear to be the same after any route of exposure, the actual toxicity of the botulinum toxins is less by inhalation.

Membrane-damaging Toxins

While neurotoxins effectively stop nerve and muscle function without causing microscopic damage to the tissues, membrane-damaging toxins destroy or damage tissue directly. For these toxins, prophylaxis is important because the point at which the pathological change becomes irreversible often occurs within minutes to a few hours after exposure.

Microcystin. An example of this type of toxin is microcystin (produced by blue-green algae), which binds covalently to a phosphatase inside liver cells; this toxin does not damage other cells of the body. Unless uptake of the toxin by the liver is blocked, irreversible damage to the organ occurs within 15 to 60 minutes after exposure to a lethal dose. When this happens, the tissue damage to the liver is so severe that therapy may have little or no value. For microcystin, unlike most toxins, the toxicity is the same no matter what the route of exposure.

Ricin. When dealing with membrane-damaging toxins, the consequences of intoxication, thus the pathogenesis of disease, may vary widely with the route of exposure, even with the same toxin. Ricin, a plant toxin, kills by blocking protein synthesis in many cells of the body, but no lung damage occurs with any exposure route except inhalation. If ricin is inhaled, as would be expected during a biological attack, microscopic damage is limited primarily to the lung, and death is caused by a mechanism different from that of injected toxin.

Furthermore, when equivalent doses of the toxin are used, a much more protective antibody must be injected to protect from inhalational exposure than from intravenous injection. Finally, although signs of intoxication may not be noted for 12 to 24 hours, microscopic damage to lung tissue begins within 8 to 12 hours or less. Irreversible biochemical changes may occur within 60 to 90 minutes after exposure, again making therapy difficult.

Trichothecene Mycotoxins. Only one class of easily produced, membrane-damaging toxins, the trichothecene mycotoxins, is dermally active. Therefore, they must be considered by standards different from those for all other toxins.

Trichothecenes can cause skin lesions and systemic illness without being inhaled and absorbed through the respiratory system.

Skin exposure and ingestion of contaminated food are the two likely routes of exposure. Nanogram quantities per square centimeter of skin cause irritation, and microgram quantities cause necrosis. If the eye is exposed, microgram doses can cause irreversible injury to the cornea. These toxins, therefore, might be dispersed as larger particles, probably visible in the air and on the ground and foliage.

In contrast to treatment for exposure to any of the other toxins, simply washing the skin with soap and water within one to three hours after exposure to the trichothecene mycotoxins will eliminate or greatly reduce the risk of illness or injury.

HOW TO PROTECT YOURSELF

As stated above, most toxins are neither volatile nor dermally active. Therefore, an aggressor would most likely attempt to present them as respirable aerosols. Toxin aerosols should pose neither a significant residual environmental threat nor remain on the skin or clothing. The typical toxin cloud would, depending on meteorological conditions, either drift with the wind close to the ground or rise above the surface of the Earth and be diluted in the atmosphere.

There may, however, be residual contamination near the munition-release point. Humans in the path of a true aerosol cloud would be exposed as the agent drifts through that area. The principal way humans are exposed to such a cloud is through breathing. Aerosol particles must be drawn into the lungs and retained to cause harm.

The protective mask, worn properly, is effective against toxin aerosols. Its efficacy, however, depends on two factors: (1) mask-to-face or hood-to-head fit and (2) use during an attack. Proper fit is vital. Because of the extreme toxicity of some of the bacterial toxins, a relatively small leak could result in a significant exposure. Eyes should be protected when possible. Definitive studies have not been done to assess the effects of aerosolized toxins on the eyes. In general, however, ocular exposure to a toxin aerosol, unless the exposed individual is near the release point, would be expected to cause few systemic effects because of the low doses absorbed.

A few toxins have direct effects on the eyes, but these are generally not toxins we would expect to be used as aerosols. Donning the protective mask prior to exposure would, of course, protect the eyes. Because important biological warfare agents are not dermally active and must be presented as respirable aerosols, special protective clothing other than the mask is less important in a toxin attack than in a chemical attack.

SPECIAL VULNERABILITIES IN CHILDREN

The release of chemical or biological toxins would disproportionately affect children through several mechanisms. With aerosolized agents (e.g., sarin, chlorine, or anthrax), the higher number of respirations per minute in children results in exposure to a relatively greater dosage. The high vapor density of gases such as sarin and chlorine places their highest concentration close to the ground in the lower breathing zone of children. The more permeable skin of newborns and children in conjunction with a larger surface-to-mass ratio results in greater exposure to transdermally absorbed toxicants. Vesicants and corrosives produce greater injury to children because of their poor skin keratinization.

Children, because of their relatively larger body surface area, lose heat quickly when showered. Consequently, skin decontamination with water may result in hypothermia unless heating lamps and other warming equipment are used. Having less fluid reserve increases the child's risk of rapid dehydration or frank shock after vomiting and diarrhea.

Finally, children have significant developmental vulnerabilities. Infants, toddlers, and young children do not have the motor skills to escape from the site of a chemical-biological incident. Even if they are able to walk, they may not have the cognitive ability to decide in which direction to flee. All children are at risk of psychological injury such as post-traumatic stress disorder from experiencing or living under the threat of chemical-biological terrorism. In a mass casualty incident, children witness injuries and deaths, possibly of their parents, which would produce both short- and long-term psychological trauma ("psychiatric casualties").

The health-care facilities responsible for treating pediatric victims in a chemical-biological event could be strained or overwhelmed. Medical facilities can become inundated with patients if large numbers of victims appear without ambulance transport and pre-entry notification. This situation differs markedly from existing hospital disaster alert systems in which victims are triaged in the field and carefully distributed among available resources to prevent any single facility from being overwhelmed.

Along similar lines, victims appearing without full hospital preparation could thwart attempts to isolate contaminated victims from other patients and hospital staff. Large-scale chemical-biological incidents necessitate the use of alternative health-care sites (e.g., auditoriums and arenas), which requires that pediatric health-care resources be dispersed to areas where victims could not receive optimal care. Injuries to health-care professionals in both office and in-hospital settings would dramatically diminish available medical resources.

Because children spend the majority of their day in school, community preparation for the chemical-biological threat should include the local educational system. Plans for rapid evacuation or the identification of in-school shelters should be established. Schools may also become a necessary site for triage and treatment of pediatric casualties, requiring that community planning include this possibility.

Children exposed to chemical or biological agents are likely to require topical decontamination by showering. Many experts suggest personal decontamination if the probability of a true exposure is high, as several infectious agents such as anthrax and smallpox can be transmitted via clothing and direct contact. When no disease has been noted but the probability of exposure is high, a reasonable approach includes showering exposed individuals and placing clothing in biohazard bags pending investigation. Removal of underclothing is not necessary.

CHAPTER FOUR

Nutritional Protection Against Bioterrorism

The tragedy that occurred on September 11, 2001, was a wake-up call that terrorism can indeed hit home. No longer is it something that is "impossible" or "inconceivable," as many once thought. One thing is certain, we are extremely fortunate that biological, chemical or radiological warfare didn't play a role in these incidents.

The Centers for Disease Control and Prevention, as a precautionary step, dispatched teams of scientists to each of the crash scenes to collect any evidence and to test for chemicals and biological agents. While we may be lucky this time, what about the next? Some people who live their lives in the precautionary spirit of "what if" will be more ready than those who believe such thoughts are too paranoid or are falling prey to conspiracy mumbo-jumbo.

A key lesson of the tragedy is that we need to

consider self-protection whenever possible. In the case of biological or radiological weapons used as tools of terrorism or mass destruction, it is likely that urban areas, as well as key political figures and members of the media, will be targeted. We have already witnessed the use of anthrax as a terrorist tool. But other weapons could include smallpox, plague, tularemia, Ebola, designer bacteria, biological toxins and dirty bombs carrying radioactive wastes that would spread upon detonation. Our nuclear plants might also be targeted.

Just as our nation must fortify its defenses against biological and other forms of terrorism, it is equally important that we fortify our own immune defenses against the same threat.

Although we hope this information will never be needed, it is important to take individual responsibility to be prepared to survive potential terrorist attacks. Lives will be saved if we put to use the information contained in this report.

IMMUNE VITALITY IS KEY TO SURVIVAL

Pathogens such as anthrax, plague, tularemia, Q fever, and brucellosis (five of the more likely agents to be used by bioterrorists) are notorious because they release lethal toxins or otherwise exert damaging effects that are simply too great for most people's immune systems to handle. For this reason, receiving proper medical management is essential. The information in this guide is not intended to replace the care of a qualified health professional.

However, even with this caveat in mind, strengthening your immunity will enable your body to put up the greatest resistance against these pathogens for the longest period possible, thus enabling you or a loved one the opportunity to survive until medical help is finally received. In case of a widespread attack, neither medical help nor the necessary drugs may be available immediately—and your body's underlying immune vitality will be key to whether you or your loved ones survive. In every case, those people with the strongest immune and antioxidant defenses will be the ones who are most likely to survive.

Dr. Ken Alibek, author of *Biohazard: The Chilling True Story of the Largest Covert Biological Weapons Program in the World—Told from Inside by the Man Who Ran It*, was born in Kauchuk, Kazakhstan, in 1950. He graduated in 1975 from the military faculty of the Tomsk Medical Institute, where he majored in infectious diseases and epidemiology. He holds a Ph.D. in microbiology for research and development of plague and tularemia biological weapons and a doctorate of science in biotechnology for developing the technology to manufacture anthrax on an industrial scale. He joined Biopreparat, the civilian arm of the biological weapons program, in 1975 and was its first deputy chief from 1988 to 1992, responsible for 32,000 employees and 40 facilities. He defected to the United States in 1992 with a personal and professional goal to make the greatest contribution he could to eliminate the danger of biological weapons.

Since his defection to the United States in 1992, he has briefed U.S. military intelligence on biological weapons. He is now working in biodefense and is president of Hadron Advanced Biosystems, which contracts with the U.S. government to develop innovative technical solutions for the intelligence community.

Recently, Advanced Biosystems was awarded a $2.6 million anthrax research contract by the U.S. Army to study and develop new medical defenses. Advanced Biosystems has also received an $800,000 grant from the National Institutes of Health to focus on very specific aspects of medical defenses against anthrax.

In a Fox News Network interview, Dr. Alibek was asked by anchor Tony Snow what people could best do to defend themselves against the threat of anthrax. **Dr. Alibek replied that the best defense at our disposal is to build a strong immune system.** *"For years," he said, " we have been talking about the importance of building a strong immune system and reducing stress."*

In a May 20, 1998 statement before the Joint Economic Committee of the U.S. Congress, Dr. Alibek, then Program Manager for the Battelle Memorial Institute, described the history, dangers, and concerns of biological weapons, including the importance of military and medical preparedness against military and terrorist attacks. In this statement he included his recommendations. Concerning the pulmonary form of anthrax caused by biological weapons, which has a high fatality rate, Dr. Alibek concluded that the usual form of antibiotic treatment is largely ineffective. He went on to say, "There are several elements in this process that can be targeted for study. The first is to find ways to modulate the immune system to counter the immunosuppressive effects of bacterial propagation in the lymph system."

In his conclusion and recommendations concerning all forms of biological threats, Dr. Alibek stated, "*Since the primary goal of developing biodefense is to save human lives, we must greatly increase our efforts to develop new treatment and urgent prophylaxis techniques. As part of this medical research,* ***we must consider a new approach in this area: fundamental research development of methods for non-specific defense, based on amplifying the immune response of the human body to invasion by any foreign agent.***

"These efforts, as well as the funds spent on research and development, will pay for themselves many times over. In addition to contributing to our nation's preparedness for a biological attack, they will provide a much-needed push in the treatment of infectious diseases that occur under natural conditions. Infectious diseases remain one of the leading causes of death in the world and cause tremendous losses, in terms of both money and human lives, every year. Furthermore, this research, especially that into methods for non-specific defense, will also contribute to the treatment of many other types of diseases, such as autoimmune disorders and cancer."

MORE BENEFITS OF BOOSTING IMMUNE FUNCTION

Even if most of us will never be challenged by bioterrorism, the benefit of insuring that one's body is experiencing optimal immune health is that we will experience fewer days of sickness due to colds or flu. Our risk of other common maladies such as heart disease and cancer (which are far more likely than a potential terrorist attack to result in death) will also be reduced. Our children especially will benefit from the nutritional information presented in this section by experiencing greater resistance to common illnesses. Let's look at our diet first and then go on to select nutritional supplements.

ADDING IMMUNE BOOSTERS TO YOUR DIET

Consume foods that traditionally support healthy immune function. Fruits, vegetables, legumes (beans) and whole grains are all sources of important antioxidant vitamins and minerals as well as fiber and other nutrients known as phytochemicals (e.g., bioflavonoids). Each of these food groups has been shown to stimulate the immune system to function optimally. Pure juices—especially vegetable juices—are also important immune-boosting beverages to consume.

Salmon, mackerel and tuna are not only low-fat protein sources, they are also, a rich source of omega-3 fatty acids, which are vital to healthy immune function. Flaxseed and flaxseed oil are rich in alpha-linolenic acid, another omega-3 fatty acid, which supports healthy immune function. We recommend Barleans' flax and products, available at health food stores.

Chicken soup contains many immune factors that help to prevent upper respiratory tract inflammation. Other soups, especially those with a mixture of spices, legumes, and vegetables, should also be consumed.

Shiitake and maitake mushrooms not only make low-fat, delectable additions to meals but are rich in beta-glucans and other proven immune boosters.

Drink green tea, as well as maitake- and ginseng-based teas.

Consume green superfoods. Chlorella, spirulina, blue-green algae, barley grass, wheat grass, and kamut will all help to boost the body's production of antibodies, which are produced by the immune cells and are responsible for disarming invading pathogens. These foods are also protective against radiation poisoning and have been used to help the children of Chernobyl recover from radiation exposure. Garden of Life's Perfect Food is an excellent green food concentrate. Mix with juice and consume daily. Contact the company at (800) 622-8986 or online at www.gardenoflife.com.

Consume iodine-rich sea vegetables, especially dietary seaweeds such as laminaria (also known as kombu), which will protect against radiation injury of the thyroid and aid in detoxification. Laminaria is rich in algin, which binds heavy metals and toxins. Equally important, its nutritious minerals, immune stimulating chains of complex polysaccharides, and natural iodine can help to displace other forms of highly toxic, radiation-contaminated iodine released from nuclear plants. Again, we refer readers to a Garden of Life formula, Living Multi, for an excellent mix of sea vegetables.

Add spices to your dishes. The white and green parts of green onion, garlic, ginger, pepper, rosemary, thyme, oregano, and mustard all possess antibacterial as well as antioxidant activity. They're great for gently boosting immune function. Add spices after cooking to avoid losing potency.

OTHER WAYS TO ENHANCE YOR IMMUNE FUNCTION

Here are some aditional ways you can enhance your immune function:

- Consider adding an under-the-sink water filter to your home. Systems utilizing activated carbon, reverse osmosis and membrane filtration can protect against some types of biological or chemical contaminants that could potentially be used to poison public water supplies.
- Be sure to wash raw produce with a mild soap. This will help to eliminate pathogens or chemicals that might be on the outer surface.
- Prefer organically grown and raised foods whenever possible. Many studies show that chronic exposure to pesticide residues has a harmful effect on immune function.
- Be wary of food service vulnerable to tampering. Salad bars, for example, are a prime example of a type of public food service that could potentially be used as a target for contamination.
- Keep up yor vitality through exercise. Exercise is highly protective against environmental toxins. If for no other reason than that exercise induces perspiration, it is extremely healthy. Studies of

human perspiration have found that the body uses its sweating mechanism to excrete heavy metals, medical and street drugs, radiation, and pesticides.

- Avoid overuse of antibiotics. By bolstering your immune function with the dietary guidelines and nutritional supplements detailed in this report, your body should be able to overcome colds or flu without needing antibiotics. Reserving the use of antibiotics for when they are really needed will enable them to be more effective.

BIOGUARD–AN IMPORTANT IMMUNE-SUPPORT FORMULA

Some of America's leading molecular scientists have been working together to develop a natural, nonprescription nutritional support formula. While by no means an anthrax cure, it may be beneficially used as a means of immune support against bioterrorism. What's more, through an innovative technology, this formula may be modified at any time to adapt to other newly emerging biological threats. This product is a long way from being labeled a cure—indeed, we don't like such terminology in the context of nutritional supplements. But you will see why we think this is critical information.

No doubt, the enemies of America would like to know the names of the scientists, their affiliations and locations in order to sabotage this research. Thus, for reasons of national security, names, locations and any other potentially identifying characteristics of these scientists have been withheld from this book.

"Normally," notes the lead scientist in this project, "when you give a person a vaccination you give them a dead or live form of the organism to produce specific antibodies." Thus when a person receives the anthrax vaccine, the body is stimulated to produce anthrax-specific antigens. Similarly, with smallpox or measles vaccines, the body produces smallpox- and measles-specific antibodies, respectively.

Starting in 1991, the lead scientist in this project began working with researchers at the Massachusetts Institute of Technology and Harvard on a method of repairing damaged and aging brain cells. "At the time," the scientist says, "I was working with cell cultures to produce neurological growth factors and bio-regulators that would heal damaged brain cells. In July of that year, however, I experienced a major breakthrough in thinking and discovered a new field of applied cell technology. It is the theory of cellular intelligence or the *smart molecule*."

This scientist had become certain that cell intelligence was comprised of even smaller subunits. He reasoned that if cells themselves have intelligence and if cells combined in animate form (as with humans and other forms of life) have intelligence, then certainly smaller units of innately intelligent life must also exist. Perhaps it is simply the biological intelligence that provides a means of survival, but it is, nonetheless, a form of intelligence.

For more than a century, science has known that bacteria, which are round, spiral, or rod-shaped single-celled microorganisms, have an innate intelligence. More recently we have learned that viruses, which are any of a large group of submicroscopic infective agents regarded either as extremely simple microorganisms or as extremely complex molecules, have innate survival intelligence. In fact, viruses, which typically contain a protein coat surrounding an RNA or DNA core of genetic material but no semipermeable membrane, are capable of growth and multiplication only in living cells. Since 1982, we have used the term *prion* for protein particles that lack nucleic acids and are believed to be the cause of various infectious diseases of the nervous system (such as bovine spongiform encephalopathy and Creutzfeldt-Jakob disease).

There are certain molecules—the scientist calls them "bions" or "smart molecules"—that can actually reproduce themselves, repair, and purify themselves, and these make up cellular life itself. "This is the fundamental regulating system in all life," says the scientist.

"WHAT DOESN'T KILL ME MAKES ME STRONGER"

It was Nietzsche who once said, "What doesn't kill me makes me stronger." What if one were to deliberately infect an organism so as to cause it to fight for its life? The dosage would not be enough to kill it but only enough to make it stronger. Let's call it training the organisms' own immunity to become stronger.

Typically, we think of this as undesirable. Take veterinary use of antibiotics. This is not so different from what the livestock industry is doing with its use of antibiotics in animal husbandry, inadvertently breeding super-strains of bacteria that, instead of dying, adapt and become even stronger.

In the case of neuro-growth factors and bioregulators, the scientists were using pseudotoxins that would place healthy murine brain cells in a defensive mode, challenging their very right to life, fertility—their very viability. "If I were to give them something overtly toxic, it would kill them outright,"says the scientist. "But I used selective toxins that, instead of killing them, challenged them to become even stronger. We caused a major resistance that stimulated these cell colonies to produce very powerful chemicals. Then I would filter off the broth through electrophoresis [which is the movement of suspended particles through a fluid or gel under the action of an electromotive force]. We used high performance chromatography to separate the broth into individual components and further characterized the individual components by their molecular weight and further *in vitro* challenges."

They took the individual components of this broth and applied them to damaged murine brain cells. "We could see regeneration and sprouting of new dendrites, the branching protoplasmic treelike strands that conduct impulses toward the body of a nerve cell," says the scientist. In a sense, he says, his team created 'Miracle Gro' for the brain. "Our research in this area is now supported through private funding and we hope that it will soon enter the clinical trial stage."

Not all of the bio-regulators were effective at neuroregeneration. Some, however, exhibited powerful antimicrobial activity. "I had friends who needed HIV treatment," says the scientist. "We found that some of the individual components were effective against HIV when we tested them *in vitro* (in the test tube) and *in vivo* (in living organisms). This is not to say that what we were doing could be termed anything like a cure. That would require human clinical data. Let's just say we demonstrated promising results.

"We found we had a whole new category of antimicrobial substances. We began developing liquid products that would be absorbed sublingually and bypass the destructive processes of the gastrointestinal tract. Word got around and intense interested was generated among scientists affiliated with MIT, Harvard, Northeastern, Tufts, Massachusetts College of Pharmacy, and Boston University. These scientists told others, and soon scientists worldwide were making appointments to receive our 'broth.'"

The scientists applied the fundamental principle of the smart molecule to a wide range of health needs. For example, by exposing cell cultures to sublethal amounts of various pathogens, protective chemicals—pathogen-specific antibodies—would be produced as a means of furthering their own survival. Taking unexposed cell cultures and exposing them to the pathogen resulted in cell death. Taking the same cell cultures and combining them with individually characterized pathogen-specific antibodies conferred protection. The cells survived exposure to the pathogens and inhibited the growth of the pathogen.

In 1993, the World Trade Center was bombed and the scientists involved in this research realized that terrorists could soon bring the war to the homeland. Thus, they intensified their research. They began inoculating cell cultures with bacterial and viral pathogens, including anthrax and smallpox cultures, that were likely to be used as weapons of bioterrorism. In fact, cells were exposed to four different anthrax strains.

"I take the infectious agent and inoculate it into a cell culture and then allow the fermentation process to proceed," says the scientist. "We then take the antibodies from this organism and isolate the active antimicrobial agents. The cells also produce other compounds that stimulate the immune system greatly. We see, for example, increased cytokines and interleukins."

Isolated components of the residue the cells produced were tested. Specific components of the residue protected cell cultures against anthrax and smallpox. Further confirmation was required. *In vivo* murine studies showed that when unprotected animals were exposed to anthrax and smallpox they died. The animals exposed to anthrax and smallpox were resistant to the pathogens when they were given *oral* doses of the specific protective isolates.

According to animal studies, the body produces more anthrax-specific immunoglobulins when given the formula—and the protection appears to last for some time even when the animals are no longer given the agent. "When you give [it to] animals with the disease, it goes away if they get the formula. We have gone as far as one year without giving them the formula and challenged animals. It has protected them."

The process may be characterized as passive immunization. But, again, we emphasize this is not a cure. No such claims are being made by the manufacturer, the scientists, or us. We have some empirical data that appear promising. We need more data, and the data needs to get published. So we want to warn anyone from thinking of this as a cure. If someone were to be stricken today with anthrax, the smart thing to do would be to first follow your doctor's instructions.

FORMULA CAN BE QUICKLY FINE TUNED

"So far," the scientist says, "the formula has worked on every pathogenic organism that we have targeted." The formulation is effective against both Gram-positive and Gram-negative bacteria. The formula is so specific in its targeted effects that it does not harm friendly bacteria. It has been tested both *in vitro* and *in vivo* against more than 500 strains of infectious microbes, including HIV, staph, strep, *E. coli* 0157 (one of the most deadly *E. coli* strains), plague, and Ebola virus. However, the technique being utilized allows the formula to be fine-tuned and modified against newly emerging pathogenic threats.

Being Used by Leading Scientists

The formula is already being used among members of the scientific community. Because this private group of highly educated scientists and academicians is working together for the good of humanity, they have decided to make this formula available to the public. "We want to help," says the lead scientist. "We think the world is in a crisis situation. We have something that is potentially powerful and safe."

The formula is called BioGuard™. It contains smart molecules isolated from the residue of specifically cultured cells. *In vivo* studies demonstrate oral absorption and efficacy. Long-term use of this formula and studies with lower life forms have shown these formulas to be safe with absolutely no untoward effects. The components of BioGuard are actually part of our normal physiology.

It would be imprudent to characterize BioGuard as an agent that can cure any disease. But it is reasonable, based on available evidence, for us to state that it appears BioGuard will support the immune system's underlying vitality and resistance—and that it may be particularly helpful against weapons of bioterrorism. Even if one gains only a few more days of resistance to deadly pathogens, this may mean the difference between life and death when additional medical help is received.

BioGuard is produced by ASN/Maxam Nutriceutics and is available at a limited number of health food stores. The company's phone number is toll-free (800) 800-9119.

IMPORTANT WHOLE-FOOD CONCENTRATES & DIETARY SUPPLEMENTS TO PROTECT AGAINST BIOTERRORISM

Inuflora

Your immune health depends heavily upon healthy gastrointestinal (GI) function. Some 75 percent of all of the antibody-producing immune cells in the body are manufactured in the GI tract.

A whole-food supplement, Inuflora® is taken from the Jerusalem artichoke tuber. Inuflora is a nondigestible, soluble fiber that selectively feeds the body's beneficial bacteria. Inuflora is a prebiotic, which is a food ingredient that is nondigestible for the human body but is fermented selectively by beneficial intestinal microflora. Thus, it stimulates the growth and activity of bacteria with beneficial consequences for health. Inuflora is able to raise the body's immune function to new heights of protection. Even when only a quarter teaspoon of Inuflora is ingested, the body's native beneficial bacterial populations can increase by 500 percent within a month.

Inuflora makes sense to health-conscious adults but is also perfect for children. One particular product Inu-lean® (which contains Inuflora) is excellent for children who especially love to eat the delicious peppermint-chocolate chewables instead of candy. Give this to your children, knowing that this so-called "candy" is affording them extra protection against environmental threats.

When children or adults use Inuflora they produce optimal amounts of antibodies—especially Immunoglobin G (IgG) antibodies, which constitute approximately 80 percent of the major antibacterial, antifungal and antiviral antibodies in the human body. Optimal IgG activity is necessary to experience optimal immune protection.

Deficiencies of IgG are found in adults and children with recurrent bacterial infections, including those associated with otitis media, sinusitus, meningitis, and respiratory infections such as chronic chest symptoms (persistent chest colds) and impaired lung function (including some cases of steroid- and antibiotic-responding asthma) as well as invasive infections in adults and children due to *S. pneumoniae* and *H. influenzae.*

When Inuflora is used with our recommended colostrum, and if passive immunity is conferred upon persons using both products, it may be possible that the body's IgG antibodies will help to inhibit anthrax spores from developing into active bacterial forms and impede early stages of infection.

Inuflora is available in tablet, powder, and chewable form. Inuflora poses no risk for untoward side effects. The usual dosage is one to fifteen grams daily.

Children usually prefer the Inuflora peppermint-chocolate chewables, which are known by the brand name Inu-lean. Adults usually use Inuflora powder and mix it with their yogurt or favorite juice or take Inuflora tablets. Inuflora is also available in a product called Inucal™, which contains calcium (since Inuflora enhances mineral absorption).

The Inuflora line is widely available at natural health centers and from health professionals. To find a source of Inuflora in your area, call Naturally Vitamins at (800) 899-4499.

Colostrum

The year 1996 marked the two hundredth anniversary of Edward Jenner's first experimental vaccination—that is, inoculation with the related cowpox virus to build immunity against the deadly scourge of smallpox. For centuries, smallpox had been the greatest killer of mankind. Now it may return with a vengeance if obtained and released by terrorists.

As touched on earlier, Dr. Jenner knew of the belief of country people that milkmaids who caught cowpox, a mild disease of cows characterized by pustular eruptions on the udders and teats, would never catch smallpox.[4] He reasoned that if he could inoculate a person with cowpox, he could protect them from smallpox. Finally, in 1796, Dr. Jenner vaccinated a local boy, James Phipps, with cowpox taken from a milkmaid and showed that the boy was then immune to smallpox.

Colostrum is most probably a source of similar protective factors. We don't think of colostrum as a dietary supplement. Rather, it is a whole food—a whole food concentrate. Colostrum is nature's "first food." It is the perfectly balanced "first meal" that every mammal gives its newborn. The mother produces it for only a short period of time; yet it contains numerous compounds that stimulate and support many processes in the body, including activation of the immune system, regeneration and repair of tissues, and growth of *all* types of cells. Recent studies are showing how extremely beneficial it is for humans and animals of all ages.

The immune factors in colostrum provide protection for the newborn against bacteria, toxins, virus, and disease. They activate numerous processes that are critical to the healthy function of the immune system. They stimulate factors which heighten the overall immune response and they provide support to a developing immune system until it is ready to function on its own. These same factors can offer similar benefits to adults and children—stimulating and supporting weakened immune functions.

Many people have been impressed with the potential for "passive immunity" from colostrum—protection from bacteria and viral pathogens. And although there is some immunity "passed on" from colostrum to recipient, the most remarkable benefits from the immune factors in colostrum come from their ability to strengthen the overall immune response.

With a healthy immune system, we would not have to rely on vaccines and flu shots, which have their drawbacks and are certainly not 100 percent effective. The immune factors in colostrum build and support *all* the processes that relate to healthy immune function. With the regular addition of colostrum to the diet, most individuals report a heightened immune response—fewer colds, flu, and allergies. They also notice that when they do catch a cold, they are able to move through it much more easily.

Clearly, colostrum enhances immune function. This alone confers greater overall immune vitality, which, with proper medical care, may help to survive a bioterrorist act. But because cows may still harbor cowpox viruses or be exposed to anthrax bacteria in the soil, colostrum may also contain minute amounts of cowpox- and anthrax-specific antibodies. While such studies have yet to be confirmatory in this regard, it is reasonable to suspect that colostrum provides the passive transfer of such immune factors that may help to confer some degree of immunity upon persons who ingest this whole-food concentrate.

Researchers with the Agricultural Research Center of Finland note the immunoglobulins of bovine colostrum provide the major antimicrobial protection against microbial infections and confer a passive immunity to the newborn until its own immune system matures.[5] But they add that immunizing cows with these pathogens or their antigens can raise the concentration in colostrum of specific antibodies against pathogens. These preparations can be used to give effective specific protection against different enteric diseases. Already, such colostral immunoglobulin supplements designed for farm animals are commercially available in many countries. Also, some immune milk products containing specific antibodies against certain pathogens have been launched for human use. A number of clinical studies are currently in progress to evaluate the efficacy of immune milks in the prevention and treatment of various human infections, including those caused by antibiotic-resistant bacteria.

But in the meantime, we also know colostrum is a rich source of lactoferrin, another key protector. Lactoferrin is a mineral-binding carrier protein that attaches to available iron. Certain aerobic (grow in the presence of oxygen) bacteria, like *E. coli*, require iron to reproduce and, therefore, lactoferrin is an effective substance when operating in the presence of a specific antibody to impede the growth of some microorganisms in the gut. Since some forms of bioterrorism may involve tainting our food supply, these properties attributed to lactoferrin could be important. We also know lactoferrin inhibits viral replication.[6]

"In my work as a hematologist in the former Soviet Union, I have done some research on the topic of colostrum and anthrax," notes Leonid Ber, M.D. "I found an important point for taking colostrum in this situation. It seems that anthrax causes death when it induces septic shock primarily through the action of its lethal toxin. This toxin makes the body release enormous amount of interleukin-1 (IL-1). In an experimental study, giving animals anti-IL-1 factors protected them from toxin challenge and death. Colostrum is a source of IL-1ra (receptor antagonist), which makes a good case for using it."[7,8]

Immune-Tree Colostrum is premier first-milking colostrum. Because it is taken within the first 12 hours, low-heat processed and never defatted (in contrast to some types of imported colostrum), Immune-Tree is rich in all of colostrum's naturally occurring immune factors, including disease-specific antibodies. Immune-Tree Colostrum is widely available at natural health centers and from health professionals. Especially noteworthy are Immune-Tree strawberry chewables, which, like Inuflora, are another perfect good-for-you "candy" for our children. If you have any trouble finding a source for these colostrum products, call Immune-Tree toll-free at (888) 484-8671. Health professionals can call (800) 916-3681.

Sovereign Silver (Colloidal Silver)

In a world concerned with bioterrorism and use of bacteria, viruses, and other microorganisms to inflict mortality and morbidity upon Americans, colloidal silver has emerged as one of our best weapons. In the current climate, every family in America should have a bottle of a quality preparation (we recommend Sovereign Silver) and a nebulizer.

It's interesting that a natural agent should be among those select substances shown to be effective against anthrax and other forms of biological terrorism. Especially noteworthy is the work of John Loftus and Mark Aarons. Loftus is a consultant to CBS's *60 Minutes* and ABC's *Prime Time* and a former prosecutor with the U.S. Justice Department's Nazi-hunting unit with excellent access to top-secret CIA and NATO archives. Aarons is an internationally recognized award-winning investigative journalist. Together, they authored the extremely well-documented non-fiction work *The Secret War Against the Jews* (St. Martin's Press, 1994). According to Loftus and Aarons, building on Nazi human experimentation, by the 1950s the Soviets had developed huge stockpiles of anthrax, plague, and designer bacteria as both a defensive shield and for offensive weapons.

Based on documents collected under the U.S. Freedom of Information Act, Loftus and Aarons report on the development of a potent protector called Movidyn, within the former Czechoslovakian satellite.

"Movidyn," they write, "is a form of colloidal silver, odorless, tasteless, and cheaper to produce than chlorine disinfectants." Only one part per billion of powdered Movidyn in water had a germicidal effect. "In a study of infected wells, it completely destroyed typhus, malaria, cholera, and amoebic dysentery. Drinking containers washed in Movidyn retained their germ-fighting abilities for several weeks." Not only was Movidyn a cost-effective prophylactic for most of the waterborne diseases that infect the Third World, but to the astonishment of the Soviet military Movidyn also disinfected every germ warfare bacteria in the Soviet arsenal, even their newest designed poisons. "In other words," says Loftus and Aarons, "Movidyn was *too* good."

Because of its threat to Soviet supremacy in the area of germ warfare, the authors report, the entire Czech factory was disassembled and removed to the Soviet Union. "To this day, the Movidyn formula seems to have been suppressed from the world."

Meanwhile, in the earlier part of the twentieth century, Dr. H. Bechold reported in *Colloids in Biology and Medicine*, published long before the advent of modern antibiotics, that colloidal silver is effective against anthrax.[9]

Medical Doctor Advocates Colloidal Silver

Dr. Victor Marcial-Vega, a board-certified oncologist and director of Health Horizons Rejuvenation Clinic in Coral Gables, Florida, has treated hundreds of persons with a variety of viral and bacterial pneumonias. Colloidal silver preparations using a nebulizer that will transform the colloidal silver into a fine spray have been among the most effective of all of the available treatments. A nebulizer allows natural antibacterial agents to reach deep inside the lungs to kill harmful microorganisms. Now, in the face of the current anthrax threat launched by evildoers, Dr. Marcial-Vega believes colloidal silver can do the same with anthrax spores.

"We are constantly filtering all kinds of bacteria through our lungs," Dr. Marcial-Vega told a reporter. Normally, a healthy body is able to kill off any dangerous bacteria on its own, he explained. But in the case of illness, like pneumonia or especially lethal bacteria like anthrax, the body may need some extra help. For anthrax prevention during an acute crisis, he recommends a daily nebulizer treatment with four milliliters of colloidal silver. By following this protocol, Dr. Marcial-Vega says the body may well eliminate anthrax spores before one even knows exposure has occurred. Colloidal silver may be useful to treat cutaneous anthrax with the preparation being directly applied to the affected skin, he adds.

Colloidal Silver Protocol When Exposed to Germ Warfare or for Pneumonia, Bronchitis, or Other Respiratory Infections

Based on limited experimental and clinical evidence, colloidal silver may be beneficially used against anthrax and other weapons of bioterrorism by reducing risk of infection in the first place and by providing the body with extra help, should an infection occur. But one should not use colloidal silver instead of antibiotics. The use of colloidal silver should be used to complement antibiotics.

Since the side effects that occur with a quality colloidal silver preparation are virtually nonexistent, if we were speaking to persons in high-risk situations, during time of acute crisis such as postal workers and mail handlers as well as others who are interested in perhaps marginally increasing their resistance to such bioterrorist agents, we would tell them that to use colloidal silver is a smart thing. Sovereign Silver has a product available with an atomizer. Spray a few times in your respiratory tract and inhale.

To be truly prepared, purchase a nebulizer that will transform the colloidal silver into a fine spray. At the first sign of such an attack, pour one to two tablespoons of Sovereign Silver colloidal silver into the receptacle (without saline because it compromises the particles) and breathe in for five minutes, at least six to eight times a day. Also, take one teaspoon of colloidal silver sublingually every two hours and hold for one minute.

Sovereign Silver from Natural-Immunogenics is recommended because of its proven efficacy at very low dosages against a wide range of infectious organisms and because it has outperformed all other competitive products against which it has been tested. The preparation is available at natural health centers and from health professionals, but if you need help in finding a store or health professional in your area, call Natural-Immunogenics toll free at (888) 328-8840.

Use of colloidal silver may be especially beneficial for anyone who works in mail room.

Colloidal silver preparations are solutions with very small particles of electrically charged pure silver suspended in them. The best products contain the largest number of particles from the smallest total amount of silver.[10] When fine enough silver particles are dispersed as a colloid, they can enter bacteria and exert their biocidal effect.

PROBIOTICS–ANTHRAX PROTECTORS

During these troubling times, we recommend that readers pay special attention to gastrointestinal tract health. A healthy GI tract is essential to immune function since so many of our antibody-forming cells are manufactured there. In the case of probiotics, be sure the formula you use has been closely studied and that you know it works, and you are therefore receiving full consumer value. After all, your life may depend on such quality.

Dr. Ohhira's Original Probiotic Formula has a wealth of scientific validation to show it is highly effective—and certainly one of the world's premiere probiotic formulas today. While working in Malayasia, Iichiroh Ohhira, Ph.D., a renowned microbiologist from Japan's Okayama University, observed that many of the world's longest-lived persons consumed generous amounts of fermented foods. Dr. Ohhira also observed that overuse of antibiotics, both in veterinary and human medicine, had led to the creation of new strains of "super" bacteria that had become antibiotic-resistant.

Spurred on by his long-time passion for improving human health by insuring the presence of adequate colonies of good bacteria, Dr. Ohhira's research team selectively bred a special strain of beneficial lactic acid bacteria isolated from the Southeast Asian food delicacy tempeh. Known as *Enterococcus faecalis* TH10, preliminary studies have shown this bacterium to be highly effective against even the most deadly antibiotic-resistant bacterial strains (such as methicillin-resistant *Staphylococcus aureus*).

Effective against Anthrax?

Dr. Ohhira's Original Probiotic Formula may have other important uses in these times. Preliminary evidence indicates Dr. Ohhira's Original Probiotic Formula may well be effective against some forms of disease caused by anthrax (*Bacillus anthracis*). This stems from research showing its constituents are effective against the pathogen *Bacillus cereus*, which is classified as a member of the same genus (or family) as anthrax. *Bacillus cereus*, like its notorious relative, is a spore former whose cells appear in the shape of large rods.

Viewing the Decimation

A picture is worth a thousand words. In the following electron microscopy images, we see the devastating effect of a substance called phenyllactic acid on *Bacillus cereus*. In an *in vitro* (test-tube) experiment, *Bacillus cereus* was cultured for six hours and then phenyllactic acid was added at a concentration of one percent. Since *B. cereus* is a Gram-positive strain, normal cells are diffused, but as the bacteria begin to die, they become clustered. In this study, the bacteria began to cluster after about a little more than three hours exposure. After nearly seven hours, the cells became quite clustered and, based on electron microscopy imagery, one could see their cell walls had started to disintegrate and fall apart. But when the cells were exposed to phenyllactic acid immediately (before being cultured), they died off within 20 minutes. The "antibacterial activity of phenyllactic acid was admitted to have quite immediate effect," note the researchers. Certainly, with ingested anthrax, this effect is noteworthy. Additional studies show us that the immune-support activities of the GI tract,

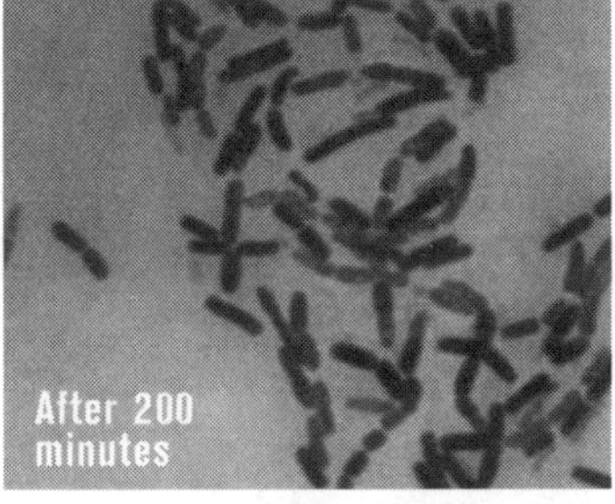

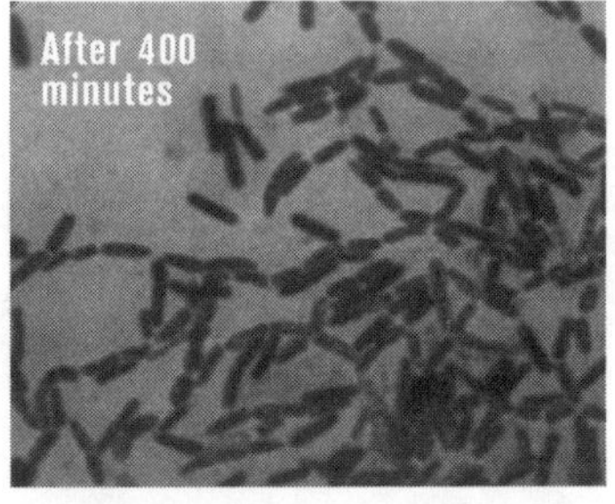

however, are systemic (i.e., occur throughout the body)—and that they may aid the body's resistance against inhalation and cutaneous anthrax.

Not only is phenyllactic acid a most potent antimicrobial compound; it is secreted by the selectively bred bacterium *Enterococcus faecalis* TH10. Fortunately, *Enterococcus faecalis* TH10 is part of Dr. Ohhira's Original Probiotic Formula. In fact, *Enterococcus faecalis* TH10 may be one of the keys to the formula's ability to subdue many of our most potent superstrains of pathogenic bacteria and to aid in the removal of toxins produced in the colon. It may also aid in survival against some of the bacterial strains that might be used by terrorists.

Dr. Ohhira's Original Probiotic Formula is made in Japan using a five-year method of manufacturing during which the special *Enterococcus faecalis* TH10 strain of bacteria, as well eleven other strains of live lactic acid bacteria, are created. The product is fermented in a natural temperature environment, during which additional raw materials are introduced, including wild herbs and fruits collected from the cold mountainous regions of the Kibi and Hiruzen Highlands of the Chugoku district of Japan as well as several species of seaweed harvested from the seas of Japan and other organic vegetables. The final formula includes 92 types of natural crops, including special leaves, bark, herbs, and fruits.

The use of *Enterococcus faecalis* TH10 in Dr. Ohhira's Original Probiotic Formula. It may well offer a degree of protection otherwise not available to most consumers. We must stress, as with all nutritional supplements, that proper medical and antibiotic therapy is necessary if you are exposed to such pathogens and this product should be used to complement their use and to help maintain vital beneficial microflora populations. The formula is now available at natural health centers and from health professionals. To have your community's health center or health professional order the formula for you, have them call Essential Formulas, Inc., at (972) 255-3918.

BETA-GLUCAN

A study, that demonstrates an orally administered particulate form of yeast beta-1,3-glucan may stimulate the immune system of mice to significantly reduce mortality from a lethal anthrax spore infection is reported in a peer-reviewed article in the *Journal of the American Nutraceutical Association* (2002; 5(2):16-20). Researchers also reported that the same orally administrated form of beta-1,3-glucan provided tumor protective effects statistically decreasing the size and weight of tumors.

Researchers at Biopolymer Engineering, Inc., Eagan, Minnesota, and from the Defence Research

Establishment Suffield (DRES), Alberta, Canada, and Biophage Pharma, Inc., Montréal, Canada, found that mice treated daily with oral, yeast-derived beta-glucan for seven days prior to injection of *Bacillus anthracis* spores had a 100 percent survival rate, compared with 50 percent for mice in the control group. The work, the authors note, is a followup to a decade of anthrax research at DRES, a center for chemical and biological defense within the Canadian Department of Defence.

"Up to now, there has been little data available concerning the efficacy of beta-1,3-glucan when taken orally," noted *JANA* editor-in-chief, Mark Houston, M.D., and associate clinical professor of medicine at Vanderbilt University School of Medicine. "This important scientific contribution demonstrates the potential benefits of this nutraceutical product against the bio-terrorism agent, anthrax (*Bacillus anthracis*)."

Numerous preclinical and clinical studies have established the anti-infective and anti-tumor properties of the beta-1,3-glucans, a natural, immune-stimulating carbohydrate, when administered by injection. The new research, according to the authors, demonstrates that these properties can be achieved with beta glucan in animals when delivered orally prior to a challenge.

The authors write that further research is needed

to "fully understand the mechanisms mediating the anthrax and tumor-protective effect. We believe that through specific interactions between the ß-1,3-glucan active component of Imucell™ WGP [beta glucan] and ß-1,3-glucan receptors on M-cells within Peyer's patches in the intestinal mucosa that a systemic signal provided by cytokines is elicited by the gut-associated lymphatic system that stimulates the innate immune system components (macrophages, neutrophils, and NK cells) to a higher functional level, increasing the first line of host defense mechanisms."

In an editorial commentary that accompanies the beta-1,3-glucan studies, *JANA* editorial board member Russell Blaylock, M.D., noted, "with the high incidence of complications associated with anthrax vaccines, an approach to protect Americans against this potential bio-terrorism agent is badly needed. Vetvicka and colleagues demonstrated in their study that the yeast derived beta-1,3-glucan given orally stimulates TNF-alpha release from the machrophage, apparently overcoming inhibition by anthrax lethal toxin. This would account for the high survival rates in the beta-1,3-glucan treated animals."

"It should be noted that while the data provided in the research by Vetvicka and colleagues is preliminary and needs to be confirmed by larger controlled trials, it is an important contribution that demonstrates the potential effectiveness of a nutraceutical product in treating infectious agents and tumors," says Dr. Bernd Wollschlaeger, assistant clinical professor of medicine and family medicine, University of Miami School of Medicine and *JANA* associate editor.

ADDITIONAL PROTECTORS

Please note that the following nutritional supplements should not be substituted for treatment in cases of germ exposure. They might, however, be used to complement your doctor's treatment.

Garlic

The Garlic Information Center in Britain indicates that anthrax is susceptible to garlic, though, again, we stress garlic should not be substituted for therapeutic treatment in cases of anthrax exposure but used only as a complement. According to the March 2001 issue of the *Journal of Nutrition*, garlic is a broad-spectrum antibiotic that even blocks toxin production by germs.

In one test garlic was found to be a more potent antibiotic than penicillin, ampicillin, doxycycline, streptomycin and cephalexin, some of the very same antibiotic drugs used in the treatment of anthrax, reports health journalist Bill Sardi, a highly rated nutritional journalist and leading expert on natural remedies. Freshly cut cloves of garlic or garlic powder may be beneficial. The antibiotic activity of one milligram of allicin, the active ingredient in garlic, equals 15 units of penicillin, notes Heinrich P. Koch, co-author of *Garlic: The Science and Therapeutic Application* (Williams & Wilkins 1996). Garlic capsules that certify their allicin content are preferred and may provide 5-10 milligrams of allicin, which is equivalent to 75-150 units of penicillin, adds Sardi. Try Garlinase® from Enzymatic Therapy, available at health food stores. Sardi recommends Allimax from Purity Products at www.purityproducts.com. (The full copyrighted Sardi report is available at www.askbillsardi.com.)

Sulfur-bearing Antioxidants

"The anthrax bacterium's toxicity emanates from its ability to kill macrophage cells which are part of the immune system," observes Sardi. "Studies have shown that sulfur-bearing antioxidants such as alpha-lipoic acid, N-acetyl cysteine, and taurine elevate levels of glutathione, a natural antioxidant within the body, which counters some of the toxicity produced by anthrax. The above sulfur compounds can be obtained from health food stores and taken in doses ranging from 100 to 500 mg."

Vitamin C

Vitamin C should be the buffered alkaline form (mineral ascorbates) rather than the acidic form (ascorbic acid) and should be combined with bioflavonoids which prolong vitamin C's action in the blood circulation, says Sardi. The powdered form of vitamin C is recommended to achieve optimal dosing. A tablespoon of vitamin C powder (about 10,000 mg) can be added to juice.

Melatonin & Dehydroepiandrosterone

Melatonin and dehydroepiandrosterone (DHEA), available at most health food stores, have been shown to help prevent lethal toxins from anthrax exposure (Shin, S. "Dehydroepiandrosterone and melatonin prevent *Bacillus anthracis* lethal toxin-induced TNF production in macrophages." *Cell Biol Toxicol* 2000;16(3):165-174).

As the researchers from the CBR Department, Agency for Defense Development, Taejon, Korea, note, "The lethal toxin of *Bacillus anthracis*, which is composed of two separate proteinaceous exotoxins, namely protective antigen and lethal factor, is central to the pathogenesis of anthrax. Low levels of this toxin are known to induce release of cytokines such as tumor necrosis factor alpha (TNF-alpha). In the present study we investigated the effect of dehydroepiandrosterone (DHEA), melatonin (MLT), or DHEA + MLT on production of lethal toxin-induced TNF-alpha in mouse peritoneal macrophages. We found that treatment with DHEA significantly inhibited the TNF-alpha production caused by anthrax lethal toxin. Exposure of MLT to anthrax lethal toxin-treated macrophages also decreased the release of TNF-alpha to the extracellular medium as compared to the control. However, combined use of DHEA and MLT also inhibited TNF-alpha release, but not more than single therapies. These results suggest that DHEA and MLT may have a therapeutic role in reducing the increased cytokine production induced by anthrax lethal toxin."

Iron and Metal-binding Chelators

"Virtually all bacteria, viruses and fungi depend upon iron as a growth factor," says Sardi. "Iron-chelating (removing) drugs and antibiotics (such as adriamycin and vancomycin), are effective against pathogens." The plague (*Yersinia pestis*), botulism, smallpox and anthrax could all be potentially treated in a complementary regimen with non-prescription metal-binding chelators, he adds. This would include colostrum (rich in lactoferrin), as well as inositol hexaphoshate (also known as IP-6 or phytic acid), which is obtained from rice bran. IP-6 has been found to have similar iron-chelating properties as desferrioxamine, a drug commonly used to kill germs, tumor cells or to remove undesirable minerals from the body, notes the September 15, 1993 issue of *Biochemistry Journal*. Enzymatic Therapy produces an excellent IP-

6 product, available at health food stores.

Oregano

The July 2001 issue of the *Journal of Food Protection* notes that oregano inhibited the growth of 25 germs such as *Staphylococcus aureas*, *Escherichia coli*, *Yersinia enterocolitica* and *Pseudomonas aeruginosa*. Purchase Oregamax™ capsules from North American Herb & Spice Co., or Fungal Defense™ from Garden of Life.

Carvacrol from oil of oregano kills spores, such as *Bacillus cereus* and *Bacillus anthracis* (anthrax), according to the October 2000 issue of the *Archives of Microbiology* and the March 1998 *Quarterly Review of Biology*.

Strengthening immune function is always important, but even more so at this time. We must be healthy to win this war.

Please remember, our recommended dietary guidelines, whole-food concentrates, and dietary supplements are not meant as a substitute for obtaining professional medical care in the event of a terrorist attack. However, our dietary guidelines and use of each of these nutritional whole-food or dietary supplements can help to strengthen the body's immune function. This may help the body to resist various potential pathogens long enough for one to survive until medical help is received.

Each formula is a superb example of immune-fortifying food concentrates and dietary supplements to be utilized during these times. Keep them handy. Use them daily, or as indicated in times of acute crisis.

CHAPTER FIVE

Nuclear and Radiation Protection

Our security services are warning that what happened on 9.11 is just the beginning, and that the next target of the terrorists will be an American nuclear facility.

In light of the recent terrorist attacks, U.S. Nuclear Regulatory Commission (NRC) officials and staff have been working around the clock to ensure adequate protection of nuclear power plants and nuclear fuel facilities. This has involved close coordination with the Federal Bureau of Investigation, other intelligence and law enforcement agencies, NRC licensees, and military, state, and local authorities.

Immediately after the attacks, the NRC advised nuclear power plants to go to the highest level of security, which they promptly did. The NRC has advised its licensees to maintain heightened security. The agency continues to monitor the situation and is prepared to make any adjustments to security measures as may be deemed appropriate.

In view of the recent unprecedented events, Chairman Richard A. Meserve, with the full support of the Commission, has directed the staff to review the NRC's security regulations and procedures.

Nuclear power plants have inherent capability to protect public health and safety through such features as robust containment buildings, redundant safety systems, and highly trained operators. They are among the most hardened structures in the country and are designed to withstand extreme events, such as hurricanes, tornadoes, and earthquakes. In addition, all NRC licensees with significant radiological material have emergency response plans to enable the mitigation of impacts on the public in the event of a release. However, the NRC did not specifically contemplate attacks by aircraft such as Boeing 757s or 767s and nuclear power plants were not designed to withstand such crashes. Detailed engineering analyses of a large airliner crash have not yet been performed.

The capacity of spent fuel dry storage casks to withstand a crash by a large commercial aircraft has not been analyzed. Nonetheless, storage casks are robust and must be capable of withstanding severe impacts, such as might occur during tornadoes, hurricanes, or earthquakes. In the event that a cask were breached, any impacts would be localized. All spent fuel storage facilities have plans to respond to such an emergency, drawn up in consultation with local officials.

There has never been an attack on a nuclear power plant. On very rare occasions there have been intrusions. For example, there was a 1993 car crash through the gates of Three Mile Island plant by an individual with a history of treatment for mental illness. Such intrusions have not resulted in harm to public health or safety.

We also face threats from "dirty" bombs containing nuclear radiation materials.

TOXIC EFFECTS FROM NUCLEAR RADIATION

Radioactive iodine (radioiodine) is a major radioisotope constituent of both nuclear power plant accidents and nuclear bomb explosions and can travel hundreds of miles on the winds.

Even very small amounts of inhaled or ingested radioiodine can do grave damage, as it will always concentrate and be retained in the small space of the thyroid gland. Eventually from such a large radiation dose to thyroid cells, abnormalities are likely to result, such as loss of thyroid function, nodules in the thyroid, or thyroid cancer. Each year 12,000 Americans discover they have thyroid cancer, though from various assorted causes, and about 1,000 die from it.

Chernobyl has shown, and continues to reveal, that the greatest danger from radioiodine is to the tiny thyroid glands of children. Researchers have found that in certain parts of Belarus, for example, 36.4 per cent of children, who were under the age of four at the time of the accident, can expect to develop thyroid cancer. This increase in incidence has been documented up to 500 kilometers from the accident site.

Health experts now estimate that the greatest health concerns affecting the largest number of people from a nuclear accident, or nuclear bomb explosion(s) anywhere in the world, will likely be from the release of radioiodine that is then carried downwind.

Going back to June 23, 1966, *The New England Journal of Medicine* (274:1442) notes: "The thyroid gland is especially vulnerable to atomic injury since radioactive isotopes of iodine are a major component of fallout."

POTASSIUM IODIDE/IODATE

Taking either potassium iodide (KI) or potassium iodate (KIO3) before exposure will saturate (fill up) a person's thyroid gland with safe stable iodine to the point where there is no room for later uptake of radioactive iodine. Once the thyroid is saturated, then any additional iodine (radioactive or stable) that is later inhaled or ingested is quickly eliminated via the kidneys.

The *bad news* is that after Three Mile Island and Chernobyl all available KI and KIO3 supplies disappeared for months, almost overnight! The KI and KIO3 market is very thin and current limited inventory will be quickly depleted in any nuclear emergency occuring anywhere in the world. (The www.ki4u.com website expects to be "out of business" within 24 hours of any nuclear emergency simply because they will be totally sold out with no illusions of getting resupplied again any time soon.)

Potassium iodide (KI) and/or potassium iodate are now being stockpiled by most developed countries for future nuclear emergencies, except for here in the United States. Very limited quantites are available for individual purchase in the United States. Radioactive iodine persists in the environment for a month or more.

Potassium iodide is much more familiar to most than they might first expect. It is the ingredient added to your table salt to make it iodized salt. Potassium iodide is approximately 76.5% iodine.

- For purposes of radiation protection, the Nuclear Regulatory Commission (NRC) states in COMSECY98016 FEDERAL REGISTER

NOTICE ON POTASSIUM IODIDE: *"In 1978, the U.S. Food and Drug Administration found KI 'safe and effective' for use in radiological emergencies and approved its over-the-counter sale."*

- Cresson H. Kearny, the author of *Nuclear War Survival Skills*, original edition published September, 1979, by Oak Ridge National Laboratory, a facility of the U.S. Department of Energy (updated and expanded 1987 edition), states on page 111: "There is no medicine that will effectively prevent nuclear radiation from damaging the human body cells that they strike. However, a salt of the elements potassium and iodine, taken orally even in very small quantities 1/2 hour to 1 day before radioactive iodines are swallowed or inhaled, prevents about 99% of the damage to the thyroid gland that otherwise would result. The thyroid gland readily absorbs both nonradioactive and radioactive iodine, and normally it retains much of this element in either or both forms."

When ordinary, nonradioactive iodine is made available in the blood for absorption by the thyroid gland before any radioactive iodine is made available, the gland will absorb and retain so much that it becomes saturated with nonradioactive iodine. When saturated, the thyroid can absorb only about one percent as much additional iodine, including radioactive forms that later may become available in the blood: then it is said to be blocked. (Excess iodine in the blood is rapidly eliminated by the action of the kidneys.)

- The Nuclear Regulatory Commission stated July 1, 1998, in USE OF POTASSIUM IODIDE IN EMERGENCY RESPONSE: *"Potassium iodide, if taken in time, blocks the thyroid gland's uptake of radioactive iodine and thus could help prevent thyroid cancers and other diseases that might otherwise be caused by exposure to airborne radioactive iodine that could be dispersed in a nuclear accident."*
- The *Federal Register* (vol. 43; Friday, December 15, 1978), states in "Potassium Iodide as a Thyroid Blocking Agent in a Radiation Emergency" that, *"almost complete (greater than 90%) blocking of peak radioactive iodine uptake by the thyroid gland can be obtained by the oral administration of ... iodide."*
- The National Council on Radiation Protection and Measurements NCRP Report No. 55. Protection of the Thyroid Gland in the Event of Releases of Radioiodine. August, 1979, states on Page 32: *"A major protective action to be considered after a serious accident at a nuclear power facility involving the release of radioiodine is the use of stable iodide as a thyroid blocking agent to*

prevent thyroid uptake of radioiodines."

- The recently updated (1999) World Health Organization (WHO) *Guidelines for Iodine Prophylaxis following Nuclear Accidents* state: *"Stable iodine administered before, or promptly after, intake of radioactive iodine can block or reduce the accumulation of radioactive iodine in the thyroid."*

Taken in time, potassium iodide (and potassium iodate, KIO3) will provide a very high level of thyroid protectio for the specific radioisotopes of iodine, which is expected by many to cause the majority of health concerns downwind from a nuclear emergency. (This is the reason most developed countries have stockpiled it.)

DOSAGE AND SAFETY OF POTASSIUM IODIDE

In April of 1982, the Bureau of Radiological Health and Bureau of Drugs, Food and Drug Administration, Department of Health and Human Services released "FINAL RECOMMENDATIONS, Potassium Iodide As A Thyroid Blocking Agent In A Radiation Emergency: Recommendations On Use." These lengthy recommendations are summarized in the FDA's "mandated patient product insert." (See below.) This insert is packed with every bottle of nonprescription potassium iodide (KI) tablets sold. However, the lengthy FDA recommendations contain many facts not mentioned in this required insert, including the following:

"Based on the FDA adverse reaction reports and an estimated 48 x 106 [48 million] 300 mg doses of potassium iodide administered each year [in the United States], the NCRP [National Council on Radiation Protection and Measurements] estimated an adverse reaction rate of from 1 in a million to 1 in 10 million doses."

(Note that this extremely low adverse reaction rate is for doses over twice as large as the 130 mg prophylactic dose.)

FDA PATIENT INFORMATION USE OF 130 MG SCORED TABLETS OF POTASSIUM IODIDE FOR THYROID BLOCKING

(Potassium Iodide Tablets, U.S.P.)
(Pronounced poeTASSeum EYEohdyed)
(Abbreviated KI)

DO NOT TAKE THIS DRUG IF YOU KNOW YOU ARE ALLERGIC TO IODINE (SEE SIDE EFFECTS BELOW).

INDICATIONS—THYROID BLOCKING IN A RADIATION EMERGENCY ONLY

DIRECTIONS FOR USE—Use only as

directed by State or local public health authorities in the event of a radiation emergency.

DOSE—*ADULTS AND CHILDREN ONE YEAR OF AGE OR OLDER:* One (1) tablet once a day. Crush for small children.

BABIES UNDER ONE YEAR OF AGE—One-half (1/2) tablet once a day. Crush first.

DOSAGE—Take for 10 days unless directed otherwise by State or local public health authorities.

Store at controlled room temperature between 15 and 30°C (59 degrees to 86 degrees F). Keep bottle tightly closed and protect from light.

WARNING—POTASSIUM IODIDE SHOULD NOT BE USED BY PEOPLE ALLERGIC TO IODIDE. Keep out of the reach of children. In case of overdose or allergic reaction, contact a physician or public health authority.

DESCRIPTION—Each (company trade name) Tablet contains 130 mg of potassium iodide.

WHO SHOULD NOT TAKE POTASSIUM IODIDE—The only people who should not take potassium iodide are people who know they are allergic to iodide. You may take potassium iodide even if you are taking medicines for a thyroid problem (for example, a thyroid hormone or anti-thyroid drug). Pregnant and nursing women and babies and children may also take this drug.

HOW AND WHEN TO TAKE POTASSIUM IODIDE—Potassium iodide should be taken as soon as possible after public health officials tell you. You should take one dose every 24 hours. More will not help you because the thyroid can "hold" only limited amounts of iodine. Larger doses will increase the risk of side effects. You will probably be told not to take the drug for more than 10 days.

SIDE EFFECTS—Usually, side effects of potassium iodide happen when people take higher doses for a long time. You should be careful not to take more than the recommended dose or take it for longer than you are told. Side effects are unlikely because of the low dose and the short time you will be taking the drug.

Possible side effects include skin rashes, swelling of the salivary glands, and "iodism" (metallic taste, burning mouth and throat, sore teeth and gums, symptoms of a head cold, and sometimes stomach upset and diarrhea).

A few people have an allergic reaction with more serious symptoms. These could be fever and joint pains, or swelling of parts of the face and body and at times severe shortness of breath requiring immediate medical attention.

Taking iodide may rarely cause overactivity of the thyroid gland, underactivity of the thyroid gland, or enlargement of the thyroid gland (goiter).

WHAT TO DO IF SIDE EFFECTS OCCUR—If the side effects are severe or if you have an allergic reaction, stop taking potassium iodide. Then, if possible, call a doctor or public health authority for instructions.

HOW SUPPLIED—Tablets (Potassium Iodide Tablets, U.S.P.): bottles of [number of tablets in a bottle] tablets. Each white, round, scored tablet contains 130 mg. potassium iodide.

While current FDA guidelines above suggest for children 1 year and older (and adults) a per day dose of 130 mg of potassium iodide (KI), the FDA is also now considering reducing the amount of the dosage for children after Chernobyl showed effective thyroid protection at even smaller doses. (This would also bring it more in line with recent World Health Organization recommendations.)

The World Health Organization's recent recommendations have a step increase in doses by age and also state the potential benefit diminishes with older adults. In fact, if only a limited number of potassium iodide (KI) or KIO3 tablets are available, these should always be given to infants, children, and young adults first, as they are the most vulnerable. Also the risk of thyroid cancer fully developing begins to drop off with adults much over 40 years of age.

The World Health Organization *Guidelines for Iodine Prophylaxis following Nuclear Accidents* state:

"In general, the potential benefit of iodine prophylaxis will be greater in the young, firstly because the small size of the thyroid means that a higher radiation dose is accumulated per unit intake of radioactive iodine. Secondly, the thyroid of the fetus, neonate and young infant has a higher yearly thyroid cancer risk per unit dose than the thyroid of an adult and, thirdly, the young will have a longer time span for the expression of the increased cancer risk."

OTHER WAYS TO DETOXIFY

There are, however, numerous other and very dangerous radioactive gases and/or types of radioactive fallout that can be associated with nuclear emergencies. Adults and children still run the risk of inhaling, ingesting, or being radiated externally from any number of dangerous nonradioiodine sources.

Here are additional detoxifying pathways:*

Spirulina (Blue-Green Microalgae)

Throughout the world now, our bodies must live within the context of low-level radiation exposures.

* Most of these detoxifying agents can be found in Perfect Food™ from Garden of Life. Call them at (800) 622-8986.

This is particularly true throughout Europe as a result of the Chernobyl disaster. We also know that our own government has consistently lied to the public about the hazards of nuclear radiation. One of the symptoms of radiation poisoning is immune dysfunction, including a high prevalence of allergic reactions characterized by high levels of Immunoglobulin E (IgE) in the blood. Such is the case for the children of Chernobyl. Those residing in highly radioactive areas have IgE levels greatly above normal.

Spirulina has demonstrated important detoxification and protective properties. Studies with 270 children show that consuming about five grams per day of spirulina tablets normalized IgE within 6 weeks.[11] Children not consuming spirulina did not experience changed IgE levels. Spirulina lowers the amount of IgE in the blood, which, in turn, normalizes and reduces allergies in the body.

We also know that radiation damages bone marrow cells. In another study, the radioprotective effect of an extract of spirulina was studied for its ability to protect bone marrow cells. The extract caused a significant reduction of gamma radiation-induced damage.[12] In a study from the Czech Republic, it was found that spirulina reduced urine radioactivity levels by 50 percent in only 20 days.[13] This result was achieved after giving five grams a day to children at the Institute of Radiation Medicine in Minsk, Belarus. The institute so believes in the purification and detoxification powers of spirulina, it has developed a program to treat 100 children every 20 days. The authors of the 1993 report conclude: "Use of spirulina decreases [radiation] dose load received from food contaminated with radionuclides, Cesium-137 and Strontium-90. Spirulina is favorable for normalizing the [adaptive] potential of children's bodies in conditions of long-lived low dose radiation."

Seaweeds

"There is no family of foods more protective against radiation and environmental pollutants than sea vegetables," says noted author Stephen R. Schecter, N.D., who wrote the highly recommended classic *Fighting Radiation & Chemical Pollutants with Foods, Herbs, & Vitamins* (Vitality Ink, 1988). Sodium alginate is thought to be one of the chemical agents in sea vegetables that is responsible for inhibition of uptake of environmental radiation and other pollutants. In 1965, it was shown that ingestion of small amounts of kelp on a daily basis was highly effective in prevention of absorption of radioactive strontium and other environmental pollutants.[14]

More recently, at the Institute of Radiation Medicine, Beijing, China, it was once again shown that sodium alginate from Laminaria species of kelp and Sargassum species of algae are highly protective.[15] Strontium absorption in human subjects was reduced by 78 percent. Ingestion completely suppressed increases of serum strontium. It was concluded that alginate preparations derived from both species are "a suitable antidote against radiostrontium absorption on a long-term basis."

At the Department of Pathology, Kitasato University School of Hygienic Sciences, Kanagawa, Japan, Drs. H. Maruyama and I. Yamamoto conducted an experiment to determine how dietary seaweeds rich in iodine and dietary fibers suppress radioactive iodine uptake by the thyroid.[16] The degree of the suppression was observed to depend on the amount of iodine in the diet. Thus, they concluded, dietary seaweeds such as kelp, which are rich in iodine and other minerals, vitamins, and beta-carotene, "may be effective in prevention of internal radiation injury of the thyroid."

Crucifers

Crucifers, rich in sulfur-containing amino acids such as cysteine and methionine, also offer some dietary protection against the effects of radiation. Researchers have found sulfur compounds bind to the membranes of cells' energy factories, mitochondria. If mitochondria are destroyed, the body's production of

The Crucifer Family

Bok choy	Kale
Broccoli	Kohlrabi
Brussels sprouts	Mustard greens
Cabbage	Radishes
Cauliflower	Red cabbage
Chinese cabbage	Rutabagas
Collards	Turnips
Horseradish	Watercress

the basic energy molecule adenosine triphosphate ceases. But when sulfur bonds to the mitochondrial membrane, cells become more resistant to radiation.[17]

One author notes: "In 1950, the researchers Lourou and Lartigue published their observations on the relationship between diet and radiation in the journal *Experientia*. They fed one group of guinea pigs cabbage and another group beets; then they exposed both groups to a dose of radiation. Later, a similar experiment was done by Spector and Calloway. One group of guinea pigs was fed just grains and [the] other [was fed] grains and cabbage. These experiment[s] found 52 percent less mortality in the cabbage group. Calloway and others repeated the experiment to test the rest of the cabbage family, including brussels sprouts, and obtained similar results."[18]

OTHER EFFECTIVE HERBS AND NUTRIENTS

Strontium 90 competes with calcium and also lowers vitamin D. Taking extra vitamin D, calcium, and magnesium plus kelp and algin, pectin and lecithin, and L-cysteine may reduce absorption and speed elimination to prevent strontium 90 from getting stored in the bones.

Several health experts have offered guidelines for protection against the effects of radiation. Paavo Airola, in *How to Get Well*, suggests a plan of high amounts of vitamin C with rutin, extra pantothenic acid, brewer's yeast, yogurt, vitamin F or essential fatty acids, inositol and lecithin, and lemon juice or lemon peel. The late Stuart Berger's guidelines in *The Immune Power Diet* include extra potassium, 1,200 mg of calcium, and 800 mg of magnesium in addition to his usual environmental protection plan of four to six grams of vitamin C, 600 IUs of vitamin E, 100 mg of zinc, and 20,000 IUs of beta-carotene. In *The Complete Guide to Anti-Aging Nutrients*, Sheldon Hendler recommends vitamins C and E, niacin, and copper to protect against the effects of x-rays and environmental toxins.

Fibers such as wheat (or oat) bran and psyllium seed husks help to increase toxin elimination.

Alfalfa, rich in chlorophylls and vitamin K, may help reduce tissue damage with radiation exposure. Apple pectin also helps bind and clear intestinal metal and chemical toxins. In *The Scientific Validation of Herbal Medicine* (Keats 1986), Daniel Mowrey, Ph.D., recommends a formula for environmental pollution including alfalfa, algin (from seaweed or algae), wheat bran, apple pectin, and kelp.

Additional herbs and nutrients known to protect against radiation include the following:

- Siberian ginseng is more properly called *eleuthero* and has been used traditionally as an immune-enhancing agent. Siberian ginseng is not really ginseng at all but a distantly related member of the ivy family. It was also employed as an anti-inflammatory, in cardiovascular disease, to restore concentration, memory, and cognition, and as a remedy for stress, depression, fatigue, or complete nervous breakdown. After the Chernobyl accident, many Russian citizens were given eleuthero to counteract the effects of radiation.
- Korean ginseng inhibits tumor cells such as sarcoma cells *in vitro*. Ginseng improves anemia and other blood deficiencies such as decreases in lymphocytes, leukcocytes, and immuloglobins, usually observed in cancer patients
- Chaparral, also known as *Larrea divaricata*, is a bitter herb that acts as a free radical scavenger. It is used for treating both bacterial and viral infections. Chaparral has been shown to protect against harmful effects of radiation and sun exposure and help prevent the formation of tumors and cancer cells in laboratory animals.

- In *Fighting Radiation and Chemical Pollutants with Foods, Herbs, and Vitamins*, Steven Schechter tells us that both black and green tea showed "radioprotective effects," whether taken before or after exposure to radiation. Among other modes of operation, tea catechins absorb radioactive isotopes and remove them from the body before they do damage. The action is similar, he says, to that of sodium alginate (the active ingredient in kelp).
- Dr. Schechter also mentions numerous research studies that document the effectiveness of aloe in preventing or treating reactions to radiation. Researchers say aloe emulsions are "recommended for treating radiation burns of the second and third degrees." In addition, "the succulent leaf of the aloe vera plant is a well-known burn remedy because it has the ability to penetrate the skin." Aloe was also found to accelerate tissue repair and normal cell growth, and to help treat other dermatological problems.
- Lecithin acts as an antioxidant and has been shown to protect against radiation and chemical pollutants by increasing high-density lipoproteins in the body.
- Cysteine, a naturally occurring amino acid, has helped counteract several kinds of radiation in animal studies in Japan and the Netherlands.

- Pectin, a carbohydrate, has been shown to help prevent assimilation of lead.
- Thymus extract, derived directly from the thymus organ, stimulates the human body to manufacture T cells.
- Charcoal and clay may be used to absorb excess radioactivity.
- Organic geranium helps to normalize calcium metabolism and is just now being studied as a potential radiation defender.

PROTECTING AGAINST BETA AND ALPHA PARTICLES

In addition to the invisible, lightlike gamma rays, fallout particles radiate two types of hazardous invisible particles: beta and alpha particles. These would pose minor dangers to informed people in fallout areas, especially to those who had entered almost any kind of shelter before the fallout began to be deposited in their area.

Beta particles are high-speed electrons given off by some of the radioactive atoms in fallout. Only the highest energy beta particles can penetrate more than about 10 feet of air or about 1/8 inch of water, wood, or human body tissue. Any building that keeps out fallout particles will prevent injury from beta radiation.

The only frequently serious dangers are from (1)

internal beta radiation doses from fallout contaminated food or drink and (2) beta burns from fresh fallout particles. Fresh fallout particles are no more than a few days old and therefore very radioactive. If fresh particles remain for at least several tens of minutes in contact with the skin, beta burns are likely to result. If only thin clothing separates fresh fallout particles from the skin, a considerably longer time will elapse before their radiation causes beta burns.

In dry, windy weather, fresh fallout particles might get inside one's nose and ears, along with dust and sand, and could cause beta burns if not promptly washed off or otherwise removed. Prompt washing will prevent beta burns. If water is not available, brushing and rubbing the fallout particles off the skin will help.

If a person is exposed outdoors where there is heavy, fresh fallout for a long enough time to receive a large dose of gamma radiation, the highest energy beta radiation given off by fresh fallout particles on the ground may be a relatively minor danger to his eyes and skin. Even ordinary glasses give good protection to the eyes against such beta radiation and ordinary clothing gives good protection to the skin.

Ordinary clothing will shield and protect the body quite well from all but the highest energy beta particles given off by fresh fallout deposited on the clothing. Fallout-contaminated clothing should be removed as soon as practical, or at least brushed and beaten before entering a shelter room, to rid it of as many fallout particles as possible. (Fallout particles that are many days old will not cause beta burns unless large quantities are on the body for hours.)

Most of the knowledge about beta burns on human skin was gathered as a result of an accident during the largest U.S. H-bomb test in the tropical Pacific. Winds blew the fallout in a direction not anticipated by the meteorologists. Five hours after the multi-megaton surface burst, some natives of the Marshall islands noticed a white powder beginning to be deposited on everything exposed, including their bare, moist skin. Unknown to them, the very small particles were fresh fallout. (Most fallout is sandlike, but fallout from bursts that have cratered calcareous rock, such as coral reefs and limestone, is powdery or flaky, and white.) Since the natives knew nothing about fallout, they thought the white dust was ashes from a distant volcanic eruption. For two days, until they were removed from their island homes and cared for by doctors, they paid practically no attention to the white dust. Living in the open and in lightly constructed homes, they received from the fallout all around them a calculated gamma ray dose of about 175 R in the two days they were exposed.

The children played in the fallout-contaminated sand. The fallout on these islanders' scalps, bare necks, and the tops of their bare feet caused itching and burning sensations after a time. Days later, beta burns resulted, along with extreme discoloration of the skin. Beta burns are not deep burns; however, it took weeks to heal them. Some, in spite of proper medical attention, developed into ulcers. (No serious permanent skin injury resulted, however.)

For survivors confined inside crowded, unsanitary shelters by heavy fallout and without medicines, beta burns could be a worse problem than were similar burns to the Marshall Islanders.

All of the Marshall Islanders unknowingly ate fallout-contaminated food and drank fallout-contaminated water for two days. Mainly as a result of this, radioactive iodine was concentrated in their thyroid glands and thyroid abnormalities developed years later.

In dry, dusty, windy areas the human nasal passages usually filter out much dust. A large part of it is swallowed and may be hazardous if the dust is contaminated with fallout. Under such dry, windy conditions, beta burns also could be caused by large amounts of dust lodged inside the nasal passages. Breathing through a dust mask, towel, or other cloth would give good protection against this localized hazard. In conclusion, persons under nuclear attack should make considerable effort to protect themselves from beta radiation.

Alpha particles, identical to the nuclei of helium atoms, are given off by some radioactive atoms in fallout. These particles have very little penetrating power: one to three inches of air will stop them. It is doubtful that alpha particles can get through unbroken skin; they cannot penetrate even a thin fabric. Alpha particles are hazardous only if materials that emit them (such as the radioactive element plutonium) enter the body and are retained in bone, lung tissue, or other parts of the body. Any shelter that excludes fallout particles affords excellent protection against this radiation danger. Unless survivors eat or drink fallout-contaminated food or water in considerably larger quantities than did the completely uninformed natives of the Marshall Islands, danger from alpha particles would be minor.

FLASH BURNS AND FLASH BLINDNESS

Flash burns are caused by the intense rays of heat emitted from the fireball within the first minute following an explosion. This thermal radiation travels at the speed of light and starts to heat or burn exposed people and materials before the arrival of the blast wave. Thermal radiation is reduced but not eliminated if it passes through rain, dense clouds, or thick smoke. On a clear day, serious flash burns on a person's exposed skin can be caused by a 20-megaton explosion that is 25 miles away.

A covering of clothing preferably of white cloth that reflects light can reduce or prevent flash burns on those who are in a large part of an area in which thermal radiation is a hazard. However, in areas close enough to ground zero for severe blast damage, the clothing of exposed people could be set on fire and their bodies badly burned.

Fires ignited by thermal radiation and those resulting from blast and other causes would especially endanger people pinned down by fallout while in or near flammable buildings.

Flash blindness can be caused by the intense light from an explosion tens of miles away in clear weather. Although very disturbing, the blindness is not permanent; most victims recover within seconds to minutes. Among the Hiroshima and Nagasaki survivors (people who had been in the open more than persons expecting a nuclear attack would be), there were a number of instances of temporary blindness that lasted as long as two or three hours, but only one case of permanent retinal injury was reported.

Flash blindness may be produced by scattered light; the victim of this temporary affliction usually has not looked directly at the fireball. Flash blindness would be more severe at night, when the pupils are larger. Retinal burns, a permanent injury, can result at great distances if the eye is focused on the fireball.

People inside any shelter with no openings through which light can shine directly would be protected from flash burns and eye damage. Persons in the open with adequate warning of a nuclear explosion can protect themselves from both flash blindness and retinal burns by closing or shielding their eyes. They should quickly get behind anything casting a shadow.

SKIN BURNS FROM HEATED DUST (THE POPCORNING EFFECT)

When exposed grains of sand and particles of earth are heated very rapidly by intense thermal radiation, they explode like popcorn and pop up into the air. While this dust is airborne, the continuing thermal radiation heats it to temperatures that may be as high as several thousand degrees Fahrenheit on a clear day in areas of severe blast. Then the shock wave and blast winds arrive and can carry the burning hot air and dust into an open shelter. Animals inside open shelters have been singed and seriously burned in some of the nuclear airburst tests in Nevada.

Thus, Japanese working inside an open tunnel shelter at Nagasaki within about 100 yards of ground zero were burned on the portion of their skin that was exposed to the entering blast wind, even though they were protected by one or two turns in the tunnel. (None of these Japanese workers who survived the blastwave effects had fatal burns or suffered serious radiation injuries, which they certainly would have suffered had they been outside and subjected to the thermal pulse and the intense initial nuclear radiation from the fireball.)

Experiments conducted during several nuclear test explosions have established the amount of thermal radiation that must be delivered to exposed earth to produce the popcorning effect. Large air bursts may result in exposed skin being burned by hot dust and heated air produced at pressure ranges as low as three or four pounds per square inch.

Protection is simple against the heated dust and very hot air that may be blown into an open shelter by the blast. When expecting an attack, occupants of an open shelter should keep towels or other cloths in hand. When they see the bright light from an explosion, they should cover their heads and exposed skin. When occupants see the very bright light from a large explosion miles away, they can close and secure such doors before the arrival of the blast wave several seconds later.

LIFE-SUPPORT EQUIPMENT FOR HEAVY FALLOUT

Shelters can be built to give excellent protection against all nuclear weapon effects, except in places within or very close to cratered areas. But most shelters would be of little use in areas of heavy fallout unless supplied with enough life-support equipment to enable occupants to stay in the shelters until conditions outside become endurable. In heavy fallout areas, most high-protection-factor shelters would be crowded; except in cold weather, most would need a ventilating pump to remove warmed air and bring in enough cooler outdoor air to maintain survivable temperature-humidity conditions. Means for storing adequate water is another essential life-support requirement.

BASEMENT SHELTERS

The blast and fire effects of a massive, all-out attack of the magnitude possible in 2003 would destroy or damage most American homes and other buildings and endanger the occupants of shelters inside them. Outside the blast and/or fire areas, the use of shelters inside buildings would not be nearly as hazardous. However, an enemy might also target some areas into which large numbers of urban Americans had evacuated before the attack.

Earth-covered expedient shelters in a blast area give better protection against injury from blast, fire, or fallout than do almost all basements. But during the more likely kinds of crises threatening nuclear war, most urban Americans, including those who would evacuate into areas outside probable blast areas, probably would lack the tools, materials, space, determination, physical strength, or time required to build good expedient shelters that are separate from buildings and covered with earth. As a result, most unprepared urban citizens would have to use basements and other shelters in existing structures, for want of better protection.

Shelters in buildings, including basement shelters, have essentially the same requirements as expedient shelters: adequate shielding against fallout radiation, strength, adequate ventilation-cooling, water, fallout radiation meters, food, hygiene, etc.

CHAPTER SIX

Protection Measures Recommended by the Department of Homeland Security

This chapter is compiled from information provided by the Department of Homeland Security.

Some of the things you can do to prepare for the unexpected, such as assembling a supply kit and developing a family communications plan, are the same for both a natural or man-made emergency. However, as you will see throughout this chapter, there are important differences among potential terrorist threats that will impact the decisions you make and the actions you take. With a little planning and common sense, you can be better prepared for the unexpected.

Terrorists are working to obtain biological, chemical, nuclear and radiological weapons and the threat of an attack is very real. At the Department of Homeland Security, throughout the federal government, and at organizations across America, experts are working hard to strengthen our nation's security. Whenever possible, we want to stop terrorist attacks before they happen. All Americans should begin a process of learning about potential threats so we are better prepared to react during an attack, notes Homeland Security Secretary Tom Ridge. While there is no way to predict what will happen, or what your personal circumstances will be, there are simple things you can do now to prepare yourself and your loved ones.

STEP 1: MAKE A KIT OF EMERGENCY SUPPLIES

Be prepared to improvise and use what you have on hand to make it on your own for *at least* three days, maybe longer. While there are many things that might make you more comfortable, think first about fresh water, food, and clean air. Consider putting together two kits. In one, put everything needed to stay where you are and make it on your own. The other should be a lightweight, smaller version you can take with you if you have to get away.

You'll need a gallon of water per person per day. Include in the kits canned and dried foods that are easy to store and prepare. If you live in a cold weather climate, include warm clothes and a sleeping bag for each member of the family.

Start now by gathering basic emergency supplies—a flashlight, a battery-powered radio, extra batteries, a first aid kit, toilet articles, prescription medicines and other special things your family may need. Many potential terrorist attacks could send tiny microscopic "junk" into the air. Many of these materials can only hurt you if they get into your body, so think about creating a barrier between yourself and any contamination. It's smart to have something for each member of the family that covers their mouth and nose.

Plan to use two to three layers of a cotton t-shirt, handkerchief or towel. Or, consider filter masks, readily available in hardware stores, which are rated based on how small a particle they filter. It is very important that the mask or other material fit your face snugly so that most of the air you breathe comes through the mask, not around it. Do whatever you can to make the best fit possible for children.

Water and Food

Water

- One gallon of water per person per day, for drinking and sanitation.
- Children, nursing mothers, and sick people may need more water.
- If you live in a warm weather climate more water may be necessary.
- Store water tightly in clean plastic containers such as soft drink bottles.
- Keep *at least* a three-day supply of water per person.

Food

- Store *at least* a three-day supply of non-perishable food.
- Select foods that require no refrigeration, preparation or cooking and little or no water.
- Pack a manual can opener and eating utensils.
- Choose foods your family will eat.
  - Ready-to-eat canned meats, fruits and vegetables
  - Protein or fruit bars
  - Dry cereal or granola
  - Peanut butter
  - Dried fruit
  - Nuts
  - Crackers
  - Canned juices
  - Non-perishable pasteurized milk
  - High energy foods
  - Vitamins
  - Food for infants
  - Comfort/stress foods

Clean Air

As mentioned, many potential terrorist attacks could send tiny microscopic particles into the air. For example, an explosion may release very fine debris that can cause lung damage. A biological attack may release germs that can make you sick if inhaled or absorbed through open cuts. Many of these agents can only hurt you if they get into your body, so think about **creating a barrier** between yourself and any contamination.

Nose and Mouth Protection

Be sure to have a supply of facemasks or dense-weave cotton material that **snugly covers your nose and mouth** and is specifically fit for each member of the family. Do whatever you can to make the best fit possible for children.

Be prepared to improvise with what you have on hand to protect your nose, mouth, eyes and cuts in your skin. Anything that fits snugly over your nose and mouth, including any dense-weave cotton material, can help filter contaminants in an emergency. It is very important that most of the air you breathe comes through the mask or cloth, not around it. Do whatever you can to make the best fit possible for children. There are also a variety of facemasks readily available in hardware stores that are rated based on how small a particle they can filter in an industrial setting.

Given the different types of attacks that could occur, there is not one solution for masking. For instance, simple cloth facemasks can filter some of the airborne "junk" or germs you might breathe into your body, but will probably not protect you from chemical gases. **Still, something over your nose and mouth in an emergency is better than nothing.** Limiting how much "junk" gets into your body may impact whether or not you get sick or develop disease.

Other Barriers

- Heavyweight plastic garbage bags or plastic sheeting
- Duct tape
- Scissors

There are circumstances when staying put and creating a barrier between yourself and potentially contaminated air outside, a process known as "**shelter-in-place**," is a matter of survival. You can use these things to tape up windows, doors and air vents if you need to seal off a room from outside contamination. Consider precutting and labeling these materials. Anything you can do in advance will save time when it counts.

Use available information to **assess the situation**. If you see large amounts of debris in the air, or if local authorities say the air is badly contaminated, you can use these things to tape up windows, doors and air vents if you need to seal off a room.

Consider also the following:

HEPA (High Efficiency Particulate Air Filtration) Filter Fans

Once you have sealed a room with plastic

sheeting and duct tape you may have created a better barrier between you and any contaminants that may be outside. However, no seal is perfect and some leakage is likely. In addition to which, you may find yourself in a space that is already contaminated to some degree.

Consider a **portable air purifier**, with a **HEPA filter**, to help remove contaminants from the room where you are sheltering. These highly efficient filters have small sieves that can capture very tiny particles, including some biological agents. Once trapped within a HEPA filter contaminants cannot get into your body and make you sick. While these filters are excellent at filtering dander, dust, molds, smoke, biological agents and other contaminants, they will not stop chemical gases.

Some people, particularly those with severe allergies and asthma, use HEPA filters in masks, portable air purifiers as well as in larger home or industrial models to continuously filter the air.

Also, include duct tape and heavyweight garbage bags or plastic sheeting that can be used to seal windows and doors if you need to create a barrier between yourself and any potential contamination outside.

Basic Supplies

- **Flashlight** and extra **batteries**
- Battery powered **radio** and extra batteries
- Plastic **garbage bags**, ties and toilet paper for personal sanitation
- **First aid kit**
- **Map** of the area for evacuation or for locating shelters
- A **whistle** to signal for help
- **Moist towelettes**
- **Clothing and Bedding**
  - If you live in a cold weather climate, you must think about warmth. It is possible that the power will be out and you will not have heat. Rethink your clothing and bedding supplies once a year to account for growing children and other family changes.
  - Have at least **one complete change of warm clothing** and shoes per person including:
    - A jacket or coat
    - Long pants
    - A long sleeve shirt
    - Sturdy shoes
    - A hat and gloves
    - A sleeping bag or warm blanket for each person.

Tools

- Emergency reference material such as a first aid book or a print out of this information
- Mess kits, or paper cups, plates and plastic utensils
- Cash or traveler's checks, change
- Non-electric can opener, utility knife
- Paper towels
- Fire extinguisher: small canister, ABC type
- Tube tent
- Pliers
- Compass
- Matches in a waterproof container
- Aluminum foil
- Plastic storage containers
- Signal flare
- Paper, pencil
- Medicine dropper
- Shut-off wrench, to turn off household gas and water
- Sanitation
- Toilet paper, towelettes
- Feminine supplies
- Personal hygiene items
- Plastic garbage bags, ties (for personal sanitation uses)
- Plastic bucket with tight lid
- Disinfectant

- Household chlorine bleach
  - You can use bleach as a disinfectant (diluted nine parts water to one part bleach), or in an emergency you can also use it to purify water. Use 16 drops of regular household liquid bleach per gallon of water. Do not use scented, color safe or bleaches with added cleaners.

Important Family Documents

Keep copies of important family records such as insurance policies, identification and bank account records in a waterproof, portable container.

BIOLOGICAL THREATS

A biological attack is the deliberate release of germs or other biological substances that can make you sick. Many agents must be inhaled, enter through a cut in the skin or be eaten to make you sick. Some biological agents, such as anthrax, do not cause contagious diseases. Others, like the smallpox virus, can result in diseases you can catch from other people.

If There is a Biological Threat...

Unlike an explosion, a biological attack may or may not be immediately obvious. While it is possible that you will see signs of a biological attack, as was sometimes the case with the anthrax mailings, it is perhaps more likely that local health care workers will report a pattern of unusual illness or there will be a wave of sick people seeking emergency medical attention. You will probably learn of the danger through an emergency radio or TV broadcast, or some other signal used in your community. You might get a telephone call or emergency response workers may come to your door.

In the event of a biological attack, public health officials may not immediately be able to provide information on what you should do. It will take time to determine exactly what the illness is, how it should be treated, and who is in danger. However, you should watch TV, listen to the radio, or check the Internet for official news including the following:

- Are you in the group or area authorities consider in danger?
- What are the signs and symptoms of the disease?
- Are medications or vaccines being distributed?
- Where?
- Who should get them?
- Where should you seek emergency medical care if you become sick?

Protect Yourself

If you become aware of an unusual and suspicious release of an unknown substance nearby, it doesn't hurt to protect yourself. Quickly get away. Cover your mouth and nose with layers of fabric that can filter the air but still allow breathing. Examples include two to three layers of cotton such as a t-shirt, handkerchief or towel. Otherwise, several layers of tissue or paper towels may help. Wash with soap and water and contact authorities.

Symptoms and Hygiene

At the time of a declared biological emergency, if a family member becomes sick, it is important to be suspicious. Do not automatically assume, however, that you should go to a hospital emergency room or that any illness is the result of the biological attack. Symptoms of many common illnesses may overlap. Use common sense, practice good hygiene and cleanliness to avoid spreading germs, and seek medical advice.

CHEMICAL THREATS

In the Case of a Chemical Threat...

A chemical attack is the deliberate release of a toxic gas, liquid or solid that can poison people and the environment.

Possible Signs of Chemical Threat

Many people suffering from watery eyes, twitching, choking, having trouble breathing or losing coordination.

Many sick or dead birds, fish or small animals are also cause for suspicion.

If You See Signs of Chemical Attack

Quickly try to **define the impacted area** or where the chemical is coming from, if possible.

Take immediate action to **get away**.

If the chemical is inside a building where you are, get out of the building without passing through the contaminated area, if possible.

Otherwise, it may be better to move as far away from where you suspect the chemical release is and "shelter-in-place."

If you are outside, quickly decide what is the **fastest escape** from the chemical threat. Consider if you can get out of the area, or if you should follow plans to "shelter-in-place."

If You Think You Have Been Exposed to a Chemical

If your eyes are watering, your skin is stinging, and you are having trouble breathing, you may have been exposed to a chemical.

If you think you may have been **exposed to a chemical, strip immediately and wash**.

Look for a hose, fountain, or any source of **water**, and wash with **soap** if possible, being sure not to scrub the chemical into your skin.

Seek emergency **medical attention**.

EXPLOSIVE THREATS

If There is an Explosion

Take shelter against your desk or a sturdy table.

Exit the building ASAP.

Do not use elevators.

Check for fire and other hazards.

Take your emergency supply kit if time allows.

If There is a Fire

- **Exit** the building ASAP.
- **Crawl** low if there is smoke
- Use a wet cloth, if possible, to **cover** your nose and mouth.
- Use the back of your hand to **feel** the upper, lower, and middle parts of closed doors.
- If the door **is not hot**, brace yourself against it and open slowly.
- If the door **is hot**, do not open it. Look for another way out.
- **Do not use** elevators.
- If you catch fire, do not run. **Stop-drop-and-roll** to put out the fire.

- If you are at home, go to a previously designated **meeting place**.
- Account for your **family** members and carefully **supervise** small children.
- **Never** go back into a burning building.

If You Are Trapped in Debris

- If possible, **use a flashlight** to signal your location to rescuers.
- **Avoid** unnecessary movement so that you don't kick up dust.
- **Cover your nose and mouth** with anything you have on hand. (Dense-weave cotton material can act as a good filter. Try to breathe through the material.)
- **Tap** on a **pipe or wall** so that rescuers can hear where you are.
- If possible, **use a whistle** to signal rescuers.
- Shout **only as** a last resort. **Shouting can cause a person to inhale dangerous amounts of dust.**

NUCLEAR BLAST THREAT

A nuclear blast is an explosion with intense light and heat, a damaging pressure wave and widespread radioactive material that can contaminate the air, water and ground surfaces for miles around. While experts may predict at this time that a nuclear attack is less likely than other types, terrorism by its nature is unpredictable.

If There is a Nuclear Blast

- **Take cover** immediately, below ground if possible, though any shield or shelter will help protect you from the immediate effects of the blast and the pressure wave.
- Quickly **assess the situation**.
- Consider if you can get out of the area or if it would be better to go inside a building and follow your plan to **"shelter-in-place."**
- In order to **limit the amount of radiation you are exposed to**, think about shielding, distance and time.
  - **Shielding:** If you have a thick shield between yourself and the radioactive materials more of the radiation will be absorbed, and you will be exposed to less.
  - **Distance:** The farther away you are from the blast and the fallout the lower your exposure.
  - **Time:** Minimizing time spent exposed will also reduce your risk.

Use **available information to assess the situation**. If there is a significant radiation threat, health care authorities may or may not advise you to take **potassium iodide**. Potassium iodide is the same stuff added to your table salt to make it iodized. It may or may not protect your thyroid gland, which is particularly vulnerable, from radioactive iodine exposure. Consider keeping potassium iodide in your emergency kit, learn what the appropriate doses are for each of your family members. Plan to **speak with your health care provider in advance** about what makes sense for your family.

DIRTY BOMB THREAT

A radiation threat or "**dirty bomb**" is the use of common explosives to spread radioactive materials over a targeted area. It is not a nuclear blast. The force of the explosion and radioactive contamination will be more localized. While the blast will be immediately obvious, the presence of radiation will not be clearly defined until trained personnel with specialized equipment are on the scene. As with any radiation, you want to try to **limit exposure**.

If There is a Radiation Threat or "Dirty Bomb"

To limit the amount of radiation you are exposed to, think about shielding, distance and time.

Shielding: If you have a thick shield between yourself and the radioactive materials more of the radiation will be absorbed, and you will be exposed to less.

Distance: The farther away you are away from the blast and the fallout the lower your exposure.

Time: Minimizing time spent exposed will also reduce your risk.

As with any emergency, local authorities may not be able to immediately provide information on what is happening and what you should do. However, you should watch TV, listen to the radio, or check the Internet often for official news and information as it becomes available.

DECIDING TO STAY OR GO

Depending on your circumstances and the nature of the attack, the first important decision is whether you stay put or get away. You should understand and plan for both possibilities. Use common sense and available information, including what you are learning here, to determine if there is immediate danger.

In any emergency, local authorities may or may not immediately be able to provide information on what is happening and what you should do. However, you should monitor TV or radio news reports for information or official instructions as they become available. If you're specifically told to evacuate or seek medical treatment, do so immediately.

Staying Put

Whether you are at home, work or elsewhere, there may be situations when it's simply best to stay where you are and avoid any uncertainty outside.

There are other circumstances when staying put and creating a barrier between yourself and potentially contaminated air outside, a process known as "shelter-in-place," is a matter of survival. Use available information to assess the situation. If you see large amounts of debris in the air, or if local authorities say the air is badly contaminated, you may want to take this kind of action.

To "Shelter-in-Place:"

- Bring your family and pets **inside**.
- **Lock** doors, **close** windows, air vents and fireplace dampers.
- **Turn off** fans, air conditioning and forced air heating systems.
- **Take your emergency supply kit** unless you have reason to believe it has been contaminated.
- **Go into an interior room** with few windows, if possible.
- **Seal** all windows, doors and air vents with plastic sheeting and duct tape. Consider measuring and cutting the sheeting in advance to save time.
- Be prepared to **improvise** and use what you have on hand to **seal gaps** so that you create a

barrier between yourself and any contamination.

- Local authorities may not immediately be able to provide information on what is happening and what you should do. However, you should **watch TV, listen to the radio or check the Internet often for official news** and instructions as they become available.

Getting Away

There may be conditions under which you will decide to get away, or there may be situations when you are ordered to leave. Plan how you will assemble your family and anticipate where you will go. Choose several destinations in different directions so you have options in an emergency.

Create an evacuation plan:

- **Plan places** where your family will meet, both within and outside of your immediate neighborhood.
- If you have a car, keep at least a **half tank of gas** in it at all times in case you need to evacuate.
- Become familiar with **alternate routes** and other means of transportation out of your area.
- If you **do not have a car**, plan how you will leave if you have to.
- **Take your emergency supply kit** unless you have reason to believe it has been contaminated.

- **Lock** the door behind you.
- Take your **pets** with you, but understand that only service animals may be permitted in public shelters. Plan how you will care for your pets in an emergency.

If time allows:

- Call or email the "out-of-state" contact in your family communications plan.
- Tell them where you are going.
- If there is damage to your home and you are instructed to do so, shut off water, gas and electricity before leaving.
- Leave a note telling others when you left and where you are going.
- Check with neighbors who may need a ride.
- Learn how and when to turn off utilities:
  - If there is damage to your home or you are instructed to turn off your utilities:
    - Locate the electric, gas and water shut-off valves.
    - Keep necessary tools near gas and water shut-off valves.
    - Teach family members how to turn off utilities.
    - If you turn the gas off, a professional must turn it back on. Do not attempt to do this yourself.

Plan for your pets:

Pets should not be left behind, but understand that only service animals may be permitted in public shelters. Plan how you will care for your pets in an emergency.

Store extra food, water and supplies for your pet.

AT WORK AND SCHOOL

Like individuals and families, schools, daycare providers, workplaces, neighborhoods and apartment buildings should all have site-specific emergency plans.

Ask about plans at the places where your family spends the most time: work, school and other places you frequent. If none exist, consider volunteering to help develop one. You will be better prepared to safely reunite your family and loved ones during an emergency if you think ahead, and communicate with others in advance.

Neighborhoods and Apartment Buildings

- A community working together during an emergency makes sense.
- **Talk to your neighbors** about how you can **work together** during an emergency.
- **Find out if anyone has specialized equipment** like a power generator, or expertise such as

medical knowledge, that might help in a crisis.

- Decide who will **check on elderly or disabled neighbors**.
- **Make back-up plans** for children in case you can't get home in an emergency.
- Sharing plans and **communicating in advance** is a good strategy.

Schools and Daycare

- If you are a parent, or guardian of an elderly or disabled adult, make sure schools and daycare providers have emergency response plans.
- Ask how they will **communicate** with families during a crisis.
- Ask if they **store** adequate food, water and other basic supplies.
- Find out if they are **prepared** to "shelter-in-place" if need be, and where they plan to go if they must get away.

Employers

- If you are an employer, make sure your workplace has a building evacuation plan that is regularly practiced.
- Take a critical look at your **heating, ventilation and air conditioning system** to determine if it is secure or if it could feasibly be upgraded to

better filter potential contaminants, and be sure you know how to turn it off if you need to.

- Think about what to do if your employees **can't go home**.
- Make sure you have appropriate **supplies** on hand.

IN A MOVING VEHICLE

- If there is an **explosion** or other factor that makes it difficult to control the vehicle, **pull over, stop the car** and **set the parking brake**.
- If the emergency could impact the physical stability of the roadway, **avoid overpasses, bridges, power lines, signs** and other hazards.
- If a power line falls on your car you are at risk of **electrical shock**, stay inside until a trained person removes the wire.
- **Listen** to the radio **for information and instructions as they become available**.

CHAPTER SEVEN

Preparing for Biological and Chemical Terrorism: A Practical Guide to Antibiotics and Their Usage for Survival

by Leonard G. Horowitz, D.M.D., M.A., M.P.H.
Tetrahedron, LLC, Sandpoint, Idaho

This document was written and posted online courtesy of Dr. Leonard G. Horowitz and Tetrahedron, LLC 206 North 4th Avenue, Suite 147, Sandpoint, Idaho 83864.

Due to the urgency of getting this information to the general public, all copyrights on the text in this chapter have been waved by Dr. Horowitz, October 1, 2000.

Antibiotics can be purchased in bulk from pharmacists or livestock and veterinarian supply stores, as well as online.

*The editors at **Healthy Living** recognize that taking antibiotics is very risky unless done under a qualified health professional's supervision. It might be good to read this piece to learn why we say this. It might be good to stock up on some of the antibiotics detailed in this book, particularly those with the broadest uses and which you or your loved ones have* *safely used before. Nevertheless, should you decide to stockpile the antibiotics detailed in this book, you should nevertheless consult a doctor when using them.*

Disclaimer and Background

This information is for educational purposes only. It is intended to help in the event of biological and chemical weapons attacks on civilian populations. It is not provided in order to diagnose or treat any disease, illness, or injury of the body, mind, or spirit.

The author, publisher, and distributors of this work accept no responsibility for people using or misusing the potentially life-saving information in this text.

Individuals suffering from any disease, illness, or injury should, as Hippocrates prescribed, "learn to derive benefit from the illness." In this sense, in the context of "America's New War" on terrorism, diagnosing the root causes of contemporary threats best derives "benefit." That is, comprehend the evil bringing on such illness and distress. The macroscopic—political, social, moral, and personal forces, beside the microscopic agents, are best identified to provide appropriate treatments.

The antibiotic applications against germ warfare discussed herein are not well-established medical practices. They are best considered speculative, but reasonable, given the urgent and widespread risks of biological attack for which there is no precedent, nor adequate scientific research. Discussions herein are intended to provide self-help strategies under emergency circumstances in which professional care is unavailable, as is anticipated following large-scale exposures of unprotected populations to lethal biologicals.

It must be stressed that the unsupervised lay use of antibiotics is dangerous for several reasons: 1) antibiotics may cause potentially fatal reactions (e.g., allergy, asthma, and death); 2) antibiotics can prompt greater growth, development, and spread of resistant pathogens such as fungi and mycoplasma prompting more severe or alternative infections; 3) antibiotic usage can make it more difficult for physicians to diagnose life-threatening infectious illnesses. Thus, self-medication is not advised under normal circumstances of medical personnel availability.

Furthermore, though certain antibiotics are customarily prescribed to kill certain strains of bacteria, germ warfare presents unique challenges. Biological weapons developers have routinely developed germ strains, such as anthrax, smallpox, influenza, mycoplasma, brucella, and more, that are antibiotic resistant. At the same time, vaccines and vaccine manufacturers have proven themselves to be highly untrustworthy.

Moreover, in the event of a biological attack, the initial benefits of antibiotic prophylaxis and treatment may be jeopardized by a second wave of infection of the same microbe, or secondary infections with other germs. These are expected due to subsequent disease transmission by infected insects, such as flies, fleas, and ticks, and immune compromised victims in which secondary infections are common.

Typically, bacteria are classified either "Gram-positive" or "Gram-negative" due to their structure and staining characteristics, which reflect their susceptibility to certain antibiotics. The penicillin family of antibiotics has been effective against Gram-positive infections. Alternatively, the tetracyclines have been used successfully to combat Gram-negative agents. These will be discussed in more detail later.

Near the beginning of a widespread biological attack, it may be extremely difficult to determine precisely the causative agent, and thereby select the proper antibiotic. This is due to: 1) the latency, or slow growth period of the germ within exposed individuals, and 2) biological weapons specialists often mix microbes to be used in such a manner as to confuse diagnosis and delay effective treatment.

For instance, a consensus of authorities predicts inhalation anthrax is among the likeliest biological weapons to be used by terrorists. This is due to its relative ease of manufacture, durability of spores, and difficulty of delayed treatment. Anthrax is a Gram-positive rod-shaped bacillus. To be more effective in killing large populations, authorities suggest that Gram-negative bacteria, such as *Pasteurella tularensis*, may accompany such attacks. This germ is likewise rod-shaped to confuse accurate diagnosis and delay time-critical treatment.

For the above reasons a "combination therapy" may be indicated and most useful in saving lives following a biological weapons attack.

WEIGHTS AND MEASUREMENTS

Safe and effective antibiotic dosages depend on accurate weights and measurements. For this reason, the following recommendations and basic knowledge is provided for lay civilians under emergency situations:

To accurately weigh antibiotics in an emergency, use the chart below. Begin by placing a ceramic cup on a postal scale. Weigh it. Next, add the powder you wish to weigh to the desired amount. For instance, if the cup alone weighs four ounces, and you require one ounce of powdered antibiotic (where, according to the chart, one ounce equals approximately thirty (30) grams, that is, thirty 1,000 milligram [mg] doses), set (or tip) the scale at five ounces with the desired antibiotic.

The same method may be used for measuring liquid doses. However, one ounce of liquid antibiotic may weigh less than once ounce on a scale. For this reason it is wise to use a graduated measuring containing, if possible, for measuring liquids.

Weights, Measures and Conversions

Solid Weights and Measures

1 ounce (oz) of solid = nearly 30 grams (gm)
1 pound (lb) = 454 grams (gm)
1 kilogram (kg) = 2.2 pounds (lb)
1 gram (gm) = 1,000 milligrams (mg)
1 grain (gr) = 64.8 mg

Liquid Weights and Measures

1 ounce (oz) of liquid = nearly 30 milliliters (ml)
1 pint = 473 ml (sometimes rounded up to 480 ml)
1 teaspoon (tsp) = 5 ml
1 tablespoon = 15 ml (that is, half [.5] an ounce)
1 milliliter (common droppers held upright) = approximately 20 drops of liquid

Antibiotic Conversions

400,000 units of penicillin = 250 milligrams (mg)

ANTIBIOTIC USAGE AND DURATION OF TREATMENT

Under normal circumstances, antibiotics are intended

to be used for approximately one to two weeks. This duration is prescribed in order to kill more slowly growing germs, such as those initially in spore forms that require incubation for disease expression.

Emergency situations may require less careful treatment durations. This is particularly true if antibiotic shortages occur as expected following a biological weapons attack. In this case, rationing may be necessary and helpful in saving more lives. ***The shortest duration of antibiotic coverage recommended following a biological attack is from the onset of symptoms to at least 72 hours after the person's symptoms completely disappear.***

Ideally, antibiotic prophylaxis (for prevention of disease) should begin as soon as a biological weapons attack is confirmed for individuals at risk of exposure. In other words, ***it is best to leave risky environments in advance of possible exposures.*** **Certainly, urban populations are at greatest risk for biological and chemical weapons attacks.**

Common Allergic Reactions to Antibiotics

Again, under normal circumstances, individuals who are hypersensitive, or allergic, to antibiotics should avoid taking them. However, following a biological weapons attack, it may warrant the risk of allergic reaction, particularly if antihistamines (such as Benadryl) are available, rather than contracting the infectious disease which is often more life-threatening. In this case, individuals who develop symptoms of allergy, including skin rashes, should ideally be under the care of a physician or hospital staff. Careful monitoring of even seemingly benign skin rashes is advised because of more urgent conditions that may result from simple allergic reactions.

Individuals with known allergies to specific antibiotics should, obviously, try to avoid taking these antibiotics. Alternative antibiotics, in this case, should be sought and used. For example, people allergic to penicillin may be able to effectively substitute erythromycin.

As detailed below, there are several types of penicillin, all of which may cause severe allergies and fatal reactions. Penicillin G and penicillin V have been known to cause more severe reactions than ampicillin. Similarly, penicillin injections have been known to cause more severe reactions than similar doses taken orally.

Approximately ten percent of people allergic to penicillin are also allergic to the cephalosporin antibiotics. The good news is that the incidence of deadly reactions to the entire class of cephalosporin antibiotics is very low.

In some liquid penicillins, manufacturers mix the anesthetic procaine (i.e., Novocain) into their formulas. Therefore, persons allergic to this commonly used dental anesthetic should avoid taking liquid penicillin suspensions.

The antibiotics suggested below for use in case of bioterrorism or biowarfare do not contain sulfur or "sulfa" drugs to which many people are allergic.

PREVENTIVE FORESIGHT REGARDING PHARMACEUTICAL SUPPLIES

The likeliest source of breaking news concerning a biological or chemical attack, launched by terrorists or other foes, is the mainstream media. By the time you hear such reports, it is likely that hospital emergency rooms, and doctor's offices, will be full of ailing victims. It typically takes a day or longer for symptoms of infectious diseases to manifest. The first signs and symptoms of a covert attack include inexplicable headaches and flu-like symptoms.

Such is the case with anthrax. The first indication of an anthrax attack, providing the strain had not been modified, is cattle becoming sick and dying. This can happen in a matter of hours. Moreover, this is an indication to begin antibiotic prophylaxis.

Under such trying circumstances, you can expect there to be tremendous demand for medical supplies and pharmaceuticals in the wake of a terrorist attack. It is, therefore, highly advisable to consider beforehand what medical supplies might be essential for your survival and the protection of your loved ones.

Obviously, people on a regimen of prescription drugs should stock, perhaps, a three months supply in a cool, dark, and dry closet or basement.

In case you need to leave your home or workplace in an emergency, try to plan, in advance, transporting your antibiotics and other medicinal requirements with you. Maintain access to standard emergency kits, particularly during times of possible trouble. Keeping one in your car is a good idea, providing the car doesn't overheat.

Given these constraints, *diabetics*, on the move in an emergency, should try to keep their insulin at room temperature until they are resettled. Above 80 degrees and while freezing insulin will begin to degrade.

In general, when traveling or storing antibiotics and medications in your car, be aware of extreme temperatures. Extreme heat and cold often inactivates, like insulin, many medicines.

A SIMPLIFIED GUIDE TO ANTIBIOTICS AND THEIR USES

Penicillins

The original penicillin-G (Pen G), along with more the common penicillin-V (Pen V), are used to fight gram-positive bacteria, such as anthrax. Pentids, the brand name for penicillin-G, come in 400 and 800 mg pills. Brand names for penicillin-V include V-Cillin-K and Pen Vee K. The basic Pen G may be purchased from farm and veterinary stores for far less expense than through pharmacies, though make sure you only buy the refrigerated brand. The active ingredients in the unrefrigerated variety are far lower and potentially inadequate.

Pen G must be taken on an empty stomach. This is not as critical for Pen V. A dose of 250 mg (i.e., 400,000 units), for people weighing 50 pounds or more, is taken four times daily. A rule of thumb for children weighing less than 50 pounds, the dosage should be reduced by 20 percent for every 10 pounds of less body weight.

These penicillins are more likely to cause allergic reactions, and fatalities, than synthetic penicillins such as ampicillin. Some of the allergic reactions are caused by procaine (Novocain) that is added in some Pen G formulas.

Ampicillin

Brand names of this synthetic penicillin include Principen, Omnipen, Polycillin and Totacillin. These are also affective against gram-positive microbes such as anthrax.

Dosages of ampicillin are the same prescribed for penicillin. This antibiotic should be taken, ideally, on an empty stomach.

Strains of anthrax that resist penicillin may be more susceptible to destruction by ampicillin. Also, ampicillin may be more helpful than penicillin for killing a broader spectrum of infections.

Cephalosporins

These are also effective against anthrax. One gram of cephalexin taken every six hours is recommended. Brand names for this are Keflex, Keflet and Keftab. One gram of the related cefadroxil, brand named Duricef, should be taken every twelve hours.

Erythromycin (Macrolide family of antibiotics)

Erythromycin and its relatives provide a broader spectrum of coverage than penicillins. Brand names of erythromycin are Pediamycin, Erythrocin, Eryc, EES, Ery-Tab, PCE, Ilosone, and E-Mycin. Other related antibiotics, such as clarithromycin (Biaxin) and azithromycin (Z-pak or Zithromax) may also be effective. A liquid form of erythromycin, called Gallimycin, is available for injection. The oral dose of this injectable product is the same.

Taken on an empty stomach, this may be used to treat more difficult cases of anthrax. If upset stomach occurs, it should be consumed with a bit of food. Avoid eating citrus fruits or products, which deactivate these antibiotics during digestion. Note:

Fatal heart attacks may result from taking these antibiotics in combination with Seldane (terfenadine), Hismanal, or Seldane-D.

For individuals weighing 150 pounds or more, a 500 mg dose is recommended. People weighing less should reduce their dosage proportionately.

Aminoglycosides

These antibiotics that are effective against anthrax, tularemia, and the Bubonic plague, include: streptomycin, gentamycin, and neomycin. They can all be extremely toxic. Primary organs at risk for destruction by the aminoglycosides include the kidneys and inner ears.

Each of the aminoglycosides must be injected, and cannot be taken orally. The oral dosage forms of these antibiotics are effective only against gastrointestinal (GI) tract infections of the stomach and intestines.

Gentamycin (Garacin) powder can be purchased in bulk. It cannot be absorbed when taken orally, but it can be effective against certain biologicals striking the GI tract such as botulism.

Streptomycin, taken two to four times daily, in one to four gram doses, equally spaced throughout the day. It can be used in combination with tetracycline until the person's fever breaks. Then the tetracycline can be continued alone. Otherwise, streptomycin should be used consistently for a week to ten days.

Gentamycin is effective against tularemia and the plague. It should be injected intramuscularly or intravenously every eight hours in emergency measures of 1.7 mg per kilogram body weight. As soon as symptoms of disease disappear, the dose should be reduced to 1.0 mg per kilogram of body weight for the remaining seven to ten day period.

This antibiotic is available in bulk through veterinary stores. It is likely that this less expensive product may be successfully used orally to defend against the plague or tularemia germs infecting the gut.

Neomycin, when given in doses of 500 mg, four times daily, may be helpful against anthrax, plague, and tularemia, though it has not been traditionally prescribed for these. Use this only if the other aminoglycoside antibiotics are unavailable.

Fluoroquinolones

In daily doses of 300 mg per kg of body weight (i.e., 65 mg per pound), ciproflavoxin (Cipro) is effective against tularemia and anthrax. The daily dose should be divided into four doses taken every six hours for two weeks. Following the terrorist attacks on September 11, 2001 on the Pentagon and World Trade Center, this extremely expensive drug has been in high demand as the FDA's antibiotic of choice against anthrax.

Chloramphenicol

Effective against anthrax, tularemia and plague, chloramphenicol (Chloromycetin) has a relatively high rate of lethal side effects. Thus, persons allergic to safer antibiotics should only use it, or in the event other medications are unavailable. More expensive than other antibiotics, this injectable product can also be consumed orally and absorbed effectively into the bloodstream. Ideally, taken on an empty stomach, it may be consumed with food to reduce stomach upsets.

Chloramphenicol has the same spectrum of activity as erythromycin. Thus, it should never be given with erythromycin unless under emergency conditions at the first sign of biowarfare-induced illness. It may, however, be taken with tetracycline for a broader spectrum of effectiveness. This combination may be wise if it is unclear which biological weapon is causing illness, and if rationing is not in effect.

The injectable form of chloramphenicol tastes awful! For people weighing 200 pounds or more, 2,500 mg doses recommended.

Tetracyclines

Tetracyclines (brand named Sumycin and Achromycin-V) are broad-spectrum antibiotics available from farm supply shops and veterinary stores in the form of oxytetracycline. These can be used effectively against most strains of anthrax, plague, and tularemia.

Oxytetracycline comes in bulk powder form under the brand name Terramycin-343. It also comes in combination with livestock feed (Advance Calf Medic). This could be used in a pinch if other antibiotics were unavailable. There are three grams of active antibiotic in each pound of feed. A low dose could be provided by consuming almost 1.5 ounces; a high dose twice that could be measured and eaten.

Two newer classes of tetracycline are doxycycline and minocycline . Brand names for these tetracyclines include the doxycyclines—Vibramycin, Vibratabs, Monodox and Doryx; and, for the minocyclines, Minocin.

Tetracycline is typically taken four times a day, doxycyclines once per day or twice per day when taken with minocycline. The two newer cyclines can be taken with food, not the older tetracycline. They, thus, tend to cause fewer stomach upsets. Doxycycline is typically less costly than traditional tetracycline, and doxycycline and minocycline provide a broader spectrum of antibiotic effectiveness than the old standard. Stains of biological weapons the may have been manufactured to resist tetracycline might be more susceptible to the newer cyclones.

As a rule of thumb, four 250 mg doses of tetracycline are prescribed daily, that is, one dose every six hours for your typical 100-pound person. For persons weighing less than 100 pound, reduce this dose accordingly. For instance, if a 100-pound person receives 1,000 mg per day, then a 50-pound person would receive 500 mg per day, or four 125 mg doses q. 6 hours. The doxycycline dosage is typically 200 mg the first day, and 100 mg doses following for up to ten days. The oxytetracycline (Terramycin) dose is the same as standard tetracycline. Another alternative tetracycline, called demeclocycline (Declomycin), may be substituted for standard tetracycline employing the same dose schedule as well.

Preserving and Administering Your Antibiotics

Most antibiotics and drugs can be preserved by refrigeration, so long as they are kept dry. If traveling through extreme temperatures, antibiotics should be encased in Styrofoam containers, at best, and efforts should be made to avoid heat or freezing cold.

Warning: No drug should be consumed beyond its expiration date, especially Tetracycline antibiotics. Severe reactions may result from this expired antibiotic.

Antibiotics are typically administered orally or by injection. However, if the patient is comatose, the oral route may be circumvented rectally by using a plastic oral syringe available in most drugstores. This should be inserted as deeply into the rectum as possible. Use of a few drops of water, then larger amounts of cocoa butter, for dissolving the antibiotic. Cocoa butter is available in most drugstores in sticks that are melted in a jar placed in hot water. The butter is commonly used for suppositories and will hold the antibiotic for absorption better than water. Water may run out of the rectum and thereby precious antibiotic may be lost. So if water is all you have, use as little as possible to dissolve and inject the measured amount of powdered antibiotic.

Antibiotic tablets can be crushed and powdered by placing them between two napkins on a hard surface and pounding them with another flat hard object or instrument.

The absorption of active antibiotic is less, given the rectal route of administration. For this reason, the dosages should be increased to compensate.

MAINTAINING HEALTHY GUT FLORA AND IMMUNITY

Three primary factors determine the outcome of a biological attack on any one individual: 1) the quantity of germs to which the person has been exposed, 2) the "pathogenicity" or power of the germs to cause disease, which depends on the unique strain, and 3) the "host resistance." This depends on the vitality of the individual's immune system.

Obviously, in the event of a biological or chemical attack, the first two factors are largely, if not entirely, beyond the control of individuals. It is upon this liability that terrorists act. But people can make a profound difference affecting the third factor-human immunity-by making a few simple choices. The first is, maintaining a healthy gut flora.

According to scientific literature, the bacteria in the large and small intestine help digest foods, support nutrient assimilation from foods, are critical in preventing infectious diseases for a number of reasons. For instance, Lactobacilli, commonly found in healthy guts, helps prevent infections from eating foods contaminated with biologicals such as botulism. A healthy gut micro flora also helps with the elimination of harmful cholesterol, toxic chemicals, and cancer-causing compounds, both natural and man-made. More than 90 percent of human immunity is, in fact, tied to lymphatic activity around the gut. Consequently, a healthy immune system is largely dependant on the intestinal flora.

Ideally, soil-based microbes, typically found on organically grown foods, should be consumed for boosting natural immunity against infectious diseases, including anthrax and other potential biological weapons. Far more effective than eating yogurt that contains Lactobacilli, there are several products available in good health food stores that supply a full pro-biotic spectrum of soil-based microbes that many alternative health professionals have been prescribing with very favorable results.

One such product is **Primal Defense** from Garden of Life. Their toll-free number is (800) 662-8986.

BIOLOGICAL WEAPONS

The following chart presents the biological weapons most likely to be used during a terrorist attack, and details concerning its diagnosis and treatment:

Agent	*Gram Staining*	*First Symptoms and Treatment*
Anthrax	positive	Headache, fever, coughing, confusion, rash, joint and muscle pain. *Treatment: tetracyclines, Pen G, ampicillin and erythromycin.*
Botulism	positive	Weakness, blurred vision, difficulty in speaking and swallowing, dry mouth, nausea, and vomiting, spreading weakness, *Treatment: Horse antitoxin*
Bubonic plague	negative	Fever, headache, abdominal distress, inability to sit or

		stand, swollen glands particularly in the groin, *Treatment: Hydration and tetracycline*
Cholera	negative	Watery diarrhea, vomiting, abdominal cramping, *Treatment: Hydration and tetracycline*
Dengue fever	parasite	Intense aching in head, muscles and joints, and fever. Second bout is accompanied by a destructive rash . *Treatment: none but symptom management.*
Ebola	virus	Headache, fever, malaise, cough, rash, and bleeding out. *Treatment: palliative*
Enterotoxin B	positive	Staphylococcus caus headache, nausea, fever and weakness. *Treatment: tetracycline, coxycycline or broad-spectrum antibiotics.*
Encephalitis	virus	Fever and headache, meningeal irritation, swollen parotid glands like mumps, skin rash with some, seizures, and brain dysfunction. *Treatment: palliative*

Smallpox	variola virus	Severe headache, high fever, skin rashes with vesicular and pustular stages of lesions. Death by secondary infections. *Treatment: palliative.*
Tularemia	negative	Fever, malaise, headache, liver swelling, ulcerating skin lesions, possible lung involvement with coughing. Treatment: streptomycin, tetracycline and chloramphenicol.

CHEMICAL WEAPONS

The following chart presents the chemical weapons most likely to be used during a terrorist attack, and details concerning diagnosis and self-aid:

Agent	***Type***	***Smell***	***Symptoms & Self-Aid***
Tubun 'GA'	Nerve	Fruity	Tightness in chest. Difficulty breathing. Runny nose. Eye pain and blurred vision. Nausea, seating, salivation, elevated pulse, heartburn, vomiting, giddiness, muscle

			spasms, involuntary urination, paralysis and respiratory arrest. *Treatment: Wash off immediately and completely. Inject two mg atropine into thigh, followed by four-gram shot of parlidoxine mesylate (oxime). If symptoms persist, give atropine again—two more two mg doses at 15-minute intervals. Apply emergency first aid, including CPR for artificial respiration for approximately two hours if breathing stops.* ***Atropine can cause serious side effects and must not be used unless there is certainty that nerve gas has caused the poisoning.***
Sarin 'GB'	Nerve	Little	Same as above.
Soman 'GD'	Nerve	Camphor	Same as above.

VX	Nerve	Unknown	Same as above.
Mustard	Blister	Garlic	Eye and skin irritant causes blistering of skin and lung damage. High risk of developing pneumonia. Symptoms delayed for up to 48 hours. Can be fatal. *Treatment: Wash off contamination immediately and completely with water. Later washes will cause worse pain. Use mydriatics, antibiotics, and local anesthetics to reduce pain. Treat blisters palliatively as burns. Bed rest.*
Phosgene	Choking	Unknown	Lung damage. Causes victim to drown in own mucous. *Treatment: Same as above.*
"CN"	Incapacitating	Blossom	Eye and skin irritant. Tearing with breathing difficulty. Nausea and headache common. *Treatment: Codeine for cough and plenty of warmth, oxygen and bed rest.*

"CS"	Incapacitating Pepper	Severe eye irritant. Causes coughing, tearing, flu-like symptoms, nausea, and breathing problems. *Treatment: Wash eyes thoroughly with warm soap and water. Breath lots of fresh air. Bed rest.*
"BZ"	Incapacitating Unknown	Skin flushes. Heart pounds irregularly with hastened pulse. Hallucination, giddiness and maniacal behavior. *Treatment: Restrain victim. Quiet bed rest.*

Notes

1 Tonduli, L.S., et al. "Effects of Huperzine used as pre-treatment against soman-induced seizures." *Neurotoxicology*, 2001;22(1):29-37.

2 Lallement, G., et al. "Efficacy of huperzine in preventing soman-induced seizures, neuropathological changes and lethality." *Fundam Clin Pharmacol*, 1997;11(5):387-394.

3 Grunwald, J., et al. "Huperzine A as a pretreatment candidate drug against nerve agent toxicity." Life Sci, 1994;54(14):991-997.

4 "Cowpox," Microsoft® Encarta® Online Encyclopedia 2000 http://encarta.msn.com © 1997-2000 Microsoft Corporation.

5 Korhonen, H., et al. "Bovine milk antibodies for health." *Br J Nutr*, 2000;84(Suppl 1):S135-S146.

6 "Antiviral effect of bovine lactoferrin saturated with metal ions on early steps of human immunodeficiency virus type 1 infection." *Int J Biochem Cell Biol*, 1998;30(9):1055-1062.

7 Hanna, P.C., et al. "On the role of macrophages in anthrax." *Proc Natl Acad Sci U S A*, 1993;90(21):10198-10201.

8 Hagiwara, K., et al. "Detection of cytokines in bovine colostrum." *Vet Immunol Immunopathol*, 2000;76(3-4):183-190.

9 Bechold, H. *Colloids in Biology and Medicine*. New York: Van Nostrand Company, 1919, pp. 368, 376.

10 Baranowski, Z. *Colloidal Silver: The Natural Antibiotic Alternative*. New York, NY: Healing Wisdom Publications, 1995.

11 Evets, L., et al. "Means to normalize the levels of immunoglobulin E, using the food supplement Spirulina," Grodenski State Medical Univ. Russian Federation Committee of Patents and Trade. Patent (19)RU (11)2005486. January 15, 1994.

12 Kolman, O.P., et al. "Radioprotective effect of extract from spirulina in mouse bone marrow cells studied by using the micronucleus test." *Toxicology Letters*, 1989; 48: 165-169.

13 Loseva, L.P. & Dardynskaya, I.V. "Spirulina—natural sorbent of radionucleides." Research Institute of Radiation Medicine, Minsk, Belarus. 6th International Congress of Applied Algology, Czech Republic, Belarus, September 1993.

14 Skoryna, S.C., et al. "Suppression of intestinal absorption of radiostrontium by substances occurring in phaeophyceae." *Proceedings of the Fifth International Seaweed Symposium*, August 25-28, 1965. Pergamonon Press, 1966: 396-397, 399.

15 Gong, Y.F., et al. "Suppression of radioactive strontium absorption by sodium alginate in animals and human subjects." *Biomed Environ* Sci, 1991; 4(3): 273-282.

16 Maruyama, H. & Yamamoto, I. "Suppression of 125I-uptake in mouse thyroid by seaweed feeding: possible preventative effect of dietary seaweed on internal radiation injury of the thyroid by radioactive iodine." *Kitasato Arch Exp Med*, 1992; 65(4): 209-216.

17 Shannon, 1993: 141.

18 Shannon, 1993: 140.